PROCEDURE CHECKLISTS TO ACCOMPANY

Fundamentals of
NURSING

Human Health and Function

Third Edition

Ruth F. Craven and Constance J. Hirnle

Elissa Swisher Sauer, MSN, RN
Assistant Dean for Health Services
Director, Nursing Programs
Reading Area Community College
Reading, Pennsylvania

Visit the Lippincott's NursingCenter Website
http://www.nursingcenter.com

Visit the Lippincott Williams & Wilkins Website
http://www.lww.com

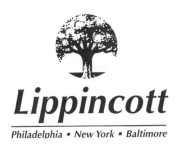

Lippincott

Philadelphia • New York • Baltimore

Ancillary Editor: Doris S. Wray
Compositor: Shepherd, Inc.
Printer/Binder: Victor Graphics

ISBN 0-7817-1912-7

INTRODUCTION

This checklist manual has been developed to provide faculty and students with a portable handbook to the procedures in the text *Fundamentals of Nursing: Human Health and Function.* These checklists may be removed and used during supervision of students' performance of procedures. They may be modified to meet the needs of the situation, if desired. Students will find these checklists helpful when reviewing for the performance of various procedures.

The procedures in the checklists follow the steps of the procedures in the book with some minor modifications. Where there are subsets of procedures—for example, measuring weight—a separate checklist is provided for each procedure. In these instances, some of the intro-

ductory steps remain the same in each procedure but the subsequent steps vary. When this occurs, the procedure step number will deviate from the checklist step number even though the content is the same. In other instances, the steps "Gather equipment," "Wash hands," "Document procedure and observations" has been added for continuity when these did not appear in the procedure in the text.

It is hoped that this manual will be useful to you, the faculty, as you teach and supervise students in the nursing classroom laboratory or in a clinical experience. It is also hoped that you, the students, will find the checklists useful in preparation for clinical experience.

LIST OF PROCEDURES

Procedure Checklists to Accompany Craven/Hirnle's Fundamentals of Nursing: Human Health and Function, third edition.

Name _____ Date _____

Unit _____ Position _____

Instructor/Evaluator _____ Position _____

Excellent ▼	Satisfactory ▼	Needs Practice ▼	**Procedure 22-1** **Measuring Weight** **Goal:** To provide baseline data from which to assess total fluid balance or nutritional status.	COMMENTS
___	___	___	1. Have client void before weighing.	
___	___	___	2. Have client wear same clothing for each weight measurement and remove slippers or shoes.	
___	___	___	3. Place protective paper or cloth on scale.	
___	___	___	4. Check that scale registers zero. Adjust as necessary.	
			Weight with Standing Scale	
___	___	___	1. Assist client onto center of scale platform. Instruct client not to lean or hold onto supports.	
___	___	___	2. Read digital display or adjust counterweights to determine client's weight.	
___	___	___	3. Assist client from scale and record weight in client's record.	
			Weight with Chair Scale	
___	___	___	1. Place scale beside client and lock wheels.	
___	___	___	2. Transfer client onto chair. If arm of chair is removable, unlock and remove before transfer. Lock back into place after transfer.	
___	___	___	3. Read digital display or adjust counterweights to determine client's weight.	
___	___	___	4. Transfer client back to bed or wheelchair.	
___	___	___	5. Clean scale according to agency policy. Return to proper location and plug in. Keep battery charged for next use.	

Excellent ▼	Satisfactory ▼	Needs Practice ▼	*Procedure 22-1* **Measuring Weight (continued)**

COMMENTS

Weight with Bed Scale

___	___	___	1. Elevate client's bed to level of stretcher scale.
___	___	___	2. With one or two assistants, turn client so that his or her back is toward the scale.
___	___	___	3. Roll scale toward bed, lock wheels in place, and lower stretcher onto bed.
___	___	___	4. Position folded stretcher under client. Roll client onto stretcher.
___	___	___	5. Attach stretcher arms to stretcher and gradually elevate stretcher about 2 inches above mattress surface. Inform client before elevating. Reassure that he or she will not fall, but the head may feel lower than the body.
___	___	___	6. Determine that stretcher is not touching any equipment. Lift drains and tubing away from stretcher.
___	___	___	7. Read digital display for client's weight.
___	___	___	8. Gradually lower stretcher to bed. Remove stretcher arms and transfer client off stretcher. Remove stretcher.
___	___	___	9. Unlock bed scale wheels and move away from bed.
___	___	___	10. Assist client to comfortable position.
___	___	___	11. Clean stretcher and scale according to agency policy.
___	___	___	12. Record weight and note any extra linen or equipment weighed with the client.

Procedure Checklists to Accompany Craven/Hirnle's Fundamentals of Nursing: Human Health and Function, third edition.

Name _____ Date _____

Unit _____ Position _____

Instructor/Evaluator _____ Position _____

Excellent ▼	Satisfactory ▼	Needs Practice ▼	*Procedure 22-2* **Assessing the Neurological System** **Goal:** To obtain baseline information about the client's neurologic status.	COMMENTS
___	___	___	1. Wash hands.	
___	___	___	2. Assemble equipment.	
			Cognitive-Sensory Assessment	
___	___	___	3. Ask direct questions requiring a verbal response to assess level of consciousness. Note appropriateness of response and emotional state.	
___	___	___	4. Evaluate client's speech patterns.	
___	___	___	5. Observe general appearance: hygiene, appropriateness of clothing to setting and to the weather.	
___	___	___	6. If responses are inappropriate, ask direct questions related to person, place, and time.	
___	___	___	7. Assess for communication or language problem.	
___	___	___	8. If client does not respond or inappropriately responds to orientation questions, give simple commands.	
___	___	___	9. If there is no response to verbal commands, test response to painful stimuli by applying firm pressure on client's sternum or finger nailbed with your thumb.	
___	___	___	10. Document level of consciousness objectively by stating specific client responses to verbal or tactile stimulation. (Use of Glasgow Coma Scale helps charting of frequent level of consciousness testing.)	
___	___	___	11. Assess function of cranial nerves:	
___	___	___	a. I (Olfactory)—Ask patient to identify different mild aromas like vanilla, coffee, chocolate, cloves.	
___	___	___	b. II (Optic)—Ask patient to read Snellen chart.	

Excellent ▼	Satisfactory ▼	Needs Practice ▼	

Procedure 22-2

Assessing the Neurological System (continued)

COMMENTS

Excellent	Satisfactory	Needs Practice	
—	—	—	c. III (Oculomotor)—Assess pupil reaction to penlight (pupillary reflex).
—	—	—	d. III—Assess direction of gaze by holding finger 18 inches from client's face. Ask client to follow finger up and down and side to side (extraocular eye movements).
—	—	—	e. IV (Trochlear)—Assess direction of gaze when testing cranial nerve II.
—	—	—	f. V (Trigeminal)—Lightly touch cotton swab to lateral sclera of eye to elicit blink.
—	—	—	g. V (con't)—Measure sensation of touch and pain on face with cotton wisp and pin.
—	—	—	h. VI (Abducens)—Assess direction of gaze when testing cranial nerve III.
—	—	—	i. VII (Facial)—Ask client to smile, frown, raise eyebrows.
—	—	—	j. VII (con't)—Ask client to identify different tastes on tip and sides of tongue: sugar, salt, lemon juice.
—	—	—	k. VIII (Auditory)—Assess ability to hear spoken word.
—	—	—	l. IX (Glossopharyngeal)—Ask client to identify different tastes on back of tongue (as in j.).
—	—	—	m. IX (con't)—Place a tongue blade on posterior tongue while client says "ah" to elicit gag response.
—	—	—	n. IX (con't)—Ask client to move tongue up and down and side to side.
—	—	—	o. X (Vagus)—Assess with cranial nerve IX by observing palate and pharynx move as client says "ah."
—	—	—	p. XI (Spinal Accessory)—Ask client to turn head side to side and shrug shoulders against resistance from examiner's hands.
—	—	—	q. XII (Hypoglossal)—Ask client to stick out tongue to midline, then move it side to side.
—	—	—	12. Assess sensory pathways (client's eyes are closed for all sensory tests):
—	—	—	a. Apply stimuli to skin in a random, unpredictable order while comparing one side of body to the other.

Excellent

Satisfactory

Needs Practice

Procedure 22-2

Assessing the Neurological System (continued)

COMMENTS

Excellent	Satisfactory	Needs Practice	
▼	▼	▼	

b. If an area of altered sensation is detected, note which spinal cord segment is affected by referring to a dermatome chart.

13. Test pain sensation first by lightly touching pointed, then blunt, end of sterile pin to proximal and distal aspects of arms and legs.

14. Test temperature sensation by touching skin with vials of hot, then cold, water.

15. Lightly stroke proximal and distal aspects of client's arms and legs with a cotton ball. Ask client to state when and where each stroke is felt.

16. Apply a vibrating tuning fork to the distal interphalangeal joint of fingers and great toe. Ask client to describe what is felt and state when it stops.

Activity-Mobility Assessment

17. Inspect arm and leg muscles for atrophy, tremors, fasiculations, or other abnormal movements.

18. Assess strength of specific muscle groups by having client extend or flex individual joints against resistance provided by examiner's hands. Test biceps, triceps, wrist and leg muscles, and ankle. Evaluate for symmetry of same muscle groups.

19. Ask client to close eyes and hold arms in front of body with palms up. Hold position for 30 seconds and observe for pronation of hands or drifting of arms.

20. Evaluate coordination and balance:

a. Have client pat upper thigh by rapidly alternating palm and back of hand.

b. With dominant hand, have client touch thumb to each finger on that hand as quickly as possible.

c. Have client use dominant forefinger to first touch your forefinger, then his or her nose repeatedly as fast as possible.

d. Romberg test—Ask client to stand with feet together, arms at sides. Have client maintain this position for 30 seconds with eyes open, then with eyes closed. Assess for swaying.

Excellent	Satisfactory	Needs Practice	

Procedure 22-2

Assessing the Neurological System (continued)

COMMENTS

—— —— —— e. Ask client to walk across room. Observe gait for symmetry, rhythm, limping, shuffling, or other abnormalities.

—— —— —— 21. Assess deep tendon reflexes (biceps, triceps, patellar, Achilles) using the following technique:

—— —— —— a. Compare symmetry of reflex on each side of body.

—— —— —— b. Extremity to be tested should be completely relaxed and slightly extended.

—— —— —— c. Hold reflex hammer loosely and allow it to swing freely into an arc.

—— —— —— d. Tap tendon briskly.

—— —— —— e. Document reflexes by grading responses 0–4+ on a stick figure, comparing bilaterally:
0–no response
1+–diminished reflex
2+–normal
3+–brisker than normal
4+–hyperactive

—— —— —— f. In newborn and infant, assess rooting, suckling, Moro, and tonic neck reflexes.

—— —— —— 22. Document all findings according to hospital policy.

Procedure Checklists to Accompany Craven/Hirnle's Fundamentals of Nursing: Human Health and Function, third edition.

Name _____ Date _____

Unit _____ Position _____

Instructor/Evaluator _____ Position _____

Excellent ▼	Satisfactory ▼	Needs Practice ▼	
			Procedure 22-3 **Auscultating Heart Sounds**
			Goal: To assess normal and abnormal functioning of the heart valves. **COMMENTS**
___	___	___	1. Wash hands.
___	___	___	2. Assist client to supine position, lifting gown to expose chest.
___	___	___	3. Warm diaphragm of stethoscope by holding between hands.
___	___	___	4. Listen in mitral area using the diaphragm. Identify first and second heart sounds. Count heart rate, noting whether rate is regular or irregular. If irregular, count for one full minute.
___	___	___	5. Listen in aortic area using the diaphragm. Concentrate first on S1, then S2, noting if splitting occurs. Listen for extra sounds.
___	___	___	6. Listen in pulmonic area still using only the diaphragm. Concentrate on S1, S2, systole, then diastole. Compare loudness of S2 in the aortic and pulmonic areas.
___	___	___	7. Move the diaphragm and listen to the tricuspid and mitral areas.
___	___	___	8. Return to aortic area. Listen in aortic area, using bell of stethoscope. Concentrate on S1, S2, systole, and diastole.
___	___	___	9. Listen, as before, in pulmonic and tricuspid areas, using bell.
___	___	___	10. Listen in mitral area, using bell. Concentrate during diastole to detect presence of a third or fourth heart sound. To increase ablility to detect a mitral murmur, have client lie on the left side while you auscultate with the bell.
___	___	___	11. Replace client's clothes. Assist to comfortable position.
___	___	___	12. Record findings describing intensity, quality, and location of sounds.

Procedure Checklists to Accompany Craven/Hirnle's Fundamentals of Nursing: Human Health and Function, third edition.

Name _____ Date _____

Unit _____ Position _____

Instructor/Evaluator _____ Position _____

Excellent	Satisfactory	Needs Practice	
▼	▼	▼	**Procedure 22-4** **Auscultating Breath Sounds** **Goal:** To assess breath sounds accurately.

COMMENTS

____	____	____	1. Wash hands.
____	____	____	2. Assemble equipment.
____	____	____	3. Assist client to upright sitting position, removing gown to expose chest.
____	____	____	4. Warm diaphragm of stethoscope by holding between hands for a short time.
____	____	____	5. Ask client to breathe deeply and slowly through mouth.
____	____	____	6. Place diaphragm of stethoscope about one inch below the middle of the right clavicle, between the ribs.
____	____	____	7. Listen for one full inspiration and exhalation on both sides of chest, noting normal and adventitious breath sounds.
____	____	____	8. Move stethoscope downward about 1.5–2 inches along midclavicular line. Note sounds on both sides of chest.
____	____	____	9. Move stethoscope downward to midclavicular line of fifth intercostal space, noting sounds on both sides of chest.
____	____	____	10. Instruct client to lean forward, crossing arms in front.
____	____	____	11. Auscultate area 2 inches below the shoulder and 2 inches to right of spine. Note sounds on both sides of chest.
____	____	____	12. Move stethoscope directly downward 2–2.5 inches. Note sounds on both sides of chest.
____	____	____	13. Repeat process. Move stethoscope downward 2–2.5 inches. Note sounds on both sides of chest.
____	____	____	14. Move stethoscope downward to area just below scapula. Note sounds on both sides of chest. Listen laterally along lower rib cage.
____	____	____	15. Replace client's clothes and assist to comfortable position.

Excellent ▼	Satisfactory ▼	Needs Practice ▼	*Procedure 22-4* **Auscultating Breath Sounds (continued)**
			COMMENTS
___	___	___	16. Discuss findings with client.
___	___	___	17. Document assessment findings, being specific as to the description and location of adventitious sounds.

Procedure Checklists to Accompany Craven/Hirnle's Fundamentals of Nursing: Human Health and Function, third edition.

Name _____ Date _____

Unit _____ Position _____

Instructor/Evaluator _____ Position _____

Excellent	Satisfactory	Needs Practice	
▼	▼	▼	**Procedure 22-5** **Auscultating Bowel Sounds**

Goal: To determine presence or absence of intestinal peristalsis.　　**COMMENTS**

Excellent	Satisfactory	Needs Practice	
____	____	____	1. Wash hands.
____	____	____	2. Warm stethoscope.
____	____	____	3. Ask client when he or she last ate.
____	____	____	4. Assist client to a supine position with abdomen exposed.
____	____	____	5. Place stethoscope diaphragm in each of the four quadrants of the abdomen. Listen for pitch, frequency, and duration of bowel sounds at each site.
____	____	____	6. If bowel sounds not heard, listen for 3–5 minutes in all quadrants before concluding that sounds are absent.
____	____	____	7. Place stethoscope bell over the epigastrum. Listen for sounds associated with pulse rate.
____	____	____	8. Proceed with rest of physical examination or cover client and assist to comfortable position.
____	____	____	9. Document findings.

Procedure Checklists to Accompany Craven/Hirnle's Fundamentals of Nursing: Human Health and Function, third edition.

Name _____ Date _____

Unit _____ Position _____

Instructor/Evaluator _____ Position _____

Excellent ▼	Satisfactory ▼	Needs Practice ▼	

Procedure 23-1
Assessing Body Temperature

Goal: To obtain baseline data for comparing future measurements or to assess for temperature alterations.

COMMENTS

Assessing Oral Temperature with Glass Thermometer

1. Wash hands. Explain procedure to client.

2. Put on disposable gloves if using a mercury thermometer.

3. Remove thermometer from storage container and rinse with cold water. Wipe dry with tissue.

4. Hold thermometer at eye level.

5. Check temperature reading on thermometer. If reading is not below 35° C, shake down by holding away from bulb between thumb and forefinger, and snap wrist sharply.

6. Place thermometer probe in client's mouth in the posterior sublingual pocket (right or left of frenulum).

7. Ask client to maintain thermometer position with lips closed.

8. Leave in place 3–5 minutes (mercury thermometer). Follow agency policy regarding recommended time interval.

9. Remove the thermometer. Wipe off secretions with tissue. Hold thermometer at eye level and rotate it slowly until mercury column is visible. Note upper end of column as temperature reading.

10. Wash mercury thermometer in soapy, tepid water. Rinse and return to storage container.

11. Record temperature on vital signs documentation record. Discuss findings with client, if appropriate.

Assessing Body Temperature (continued)

Excellent	Satisfactory	Needs Practice		COMMENTS

Assessing Axillary Temperature

1. Wash hands. Explain procedure to client.
2. Remove thermometer from storage container and rinse with cold water. Wipe dry with tissue.
3. Hold thermometer at eye level.
4. Check temperature reading on thermometer. If reading is not below 35° C, shake down by holding thermometer at end away from bulb between thumb and forefinger, and snap wrist sharply.
5. Close bedroom door or bed curtains. Assist client to comfortable position and expose axilla.
6. Insert thermometer into middle of axilla; fold client's arm down and place across chest.
7. Hold in place 9 minutes for adults; 5 minutes for children.
8. Remove the thermometer. Hold thermometer at eye level and rotate it slowly until mercury column is visible. Note upper end of column as temperature reading.
9. Wash mercury thermometer in soapy, tepid water. Rinse and return to storage container.
10. Record temperature on vital signs documentation record. Discuss findings with client, if appropriate.

Assessing Oral Temperature with Electronic Thermometer

1. Wash hands. Explain procedure to client.
2. Remove electronic thermometer from battery pack, and remove temperature probe from unit, noting digital display of temperature on screen (usually 34° C or 94° F).
3. Securely attach disposable cover over temperature probe.
4. Place and hold probe in sublingual pocket of client's mouth.
5. Wait for a beep (usually 10–20 seconds) and then remove probe from client's mouth, noting the temperature displayed on the unit.
6. Displace probe cover by pressing the probe release button as you hold the probe over a waste container.

Procedure 23-1

Assessing Body Temperature (continued)

Excellent ▼	Satisfactory ▼	Needs Practice ▼	
			COMMENTS
___	___	___	7. Return probe to storage place within the unit and the thermometer to the battery pack.
___	___	___	8. Document temperature on vital signs documentation record. Discuss findings with client, if appropriate.

**Assessing Rectal Temperature
with an Electronic Thermometer**

___	___	___	1. Wash hands. Don clean gloves and explain procedure to client.
___	___	___	2. Remove rectal (red) electronic thermometer from battery pack, and remove temperature probe from unit, noting digital display of temperature on screen.
___	___	___	3. Securely attach the disposable cover over the temperature probe.
___	___	___	4. Close bedroom door or bed curtains. Assist client to Sims's position with upper leg flexed. Expose only anal area.
___	___	___	5. Apply water-soluble lubricant liberally to thermometer probe tip.
___	___	___	6. Separate client's buttocks with one gloved hand.
___	___	___	7. Ask client to take a deep, slow breath. Insert thermometer into anus in direction of umbilicus, 1/2 inch for an infant; 1-1/2 inches for an adult. Do not force.
___	___	___	8. Hold in place until beep is heard. Obtain reading.
___	___	___	9. Displace probe cover by pressing the probe release button as you hold the probe over a waste container.
___	___	___	10. Return probe to storage place within the unit and the thermometer to the battery pack.
___	___	___	11. Record temperature on vital signs documentation record. Discuss findings with client, if appropriate.

**Assessing Temperature Using a Tympanic
Membrane Thermometer**

___	___	___	1. Remove tympanic thermometer from recharging base, and attach tympanic probe cover to sensor unit.
___	___	___	2. Insert probe into ear canal, making sure the probe fits snugly. Avoid forcing probe too deeply into ear. Pulling on pinna may help straighten ear canal, which permits better exposure of tympanic membrane. Rotate probe handle toward the jawline.

Excellent ▼	Satisfactory ▼	Needs Practice ▼	*Procedure 23-1* **Assessing Body Temperature (continued)**
			COMMENTS
——	——	——	3. Activate the thermometer and watch for the temperature readout, which is usually displayed within 2 seconds. Remove thermometer.
——	——	——	4. Eject sensor probe cover directly into waste container, and return tympanic thermometer to base for recharging.
——	——	——	5. Record temperature on vital signs documentation record. Discuss findings with client, if appropriate.

Procedure Checklists to Accompany Craven/Hirnle's Fundamentals of Nursing: Human Health and Function, third edition.

Name _____ Date _____

Unit _____ Position _____

Instructor/Evaluator _____ Position _____

Excellent)	Satisfactory	Needs Practice	
▼	▼	▼	**Procedure 23-2** **Obtaining a Pulse** **Goal:** To obtain baseline measurement of heart rate and rhythm.

COMMENTS

Obtaining a Radial Pulse

____ ____ ____ 1. Wash hands and explain procedure to client.

____ ____ ____ 2. Position client comfortably with forearm across chest or at side with wrist extended.

____ ____ ____ 3. Place fingertips of your first three fingers along the groove at base of thumb on client's wrist.

____ ____ ____ 4. Press against radial artery to obliterate pulse, then gradually release pressure until pulsations are felt.

____ ____ ____ 5. Assess pulse for regularity and strength.

____ ____ ____ 6. If pulse is not easily palpable, use Doppler:

____ ____ ____ a. Apply conducting gel to end of probe or to radial site.

____ ____ ____ b. Press "on" button and place probe against skin on pulse site. Reposition slightly using firm pressure until pulsating sound is heard.

____ ____ ____ 7. If pulse is regular, count pulse for 30 seconds and multiply by two. If pulse is irregular, count for one full minute. Initial pulse is counted as zero.

____ ____ ____ 8. Document pulse on vital signs record.

Obtaining an Apical Pulse

____ ____ ____ 1. Position client in supine or sitting position with sternum and left chest exposed.

____ ____ ____ 2. Warm diaphragm of stethoscope by holding in palm of hand for 5–10 seconds.

____ ____ ____ 3. Insert the earpieces of stethoscope into ears and place diaphragm over apex of client's heart.

____ ____ ____ 4. Assess heartbeat for regularity and dysrhythmias.

Excellent	Satisfactory	Needs Practice		
▼	▼	▼		COMMENTS
——	——	——	5. If rhythm is regular, count the heartbeat for 30 seconds and multiply by two. Count for one full minute if rhythm is irregular. Initial pulse is counted as zero.	
——	——	——	6. Replace client's gown and assist client to return to a comfortable position.	
——	——	——	7. Share results with client, if appropriate.	
——	——	——	8. Document pulse on vital signs record. Specify in documentation that an apical pulse was obtained.	

Procedure 23-2

Obtaining a Pulse (continued)

Procedure Checklists to Accompany Craven/Hirnle's Fundamentals of Nursing: Human Health and Function, third edition.

Name _____ Date _____

Unit _____ Position _____

Instructor/Evaluator _____ Position _____

Excellent	Satisfactory	Needs Practice	
▼	▼	▼	**Procedure 23-3** **Assessing Respiration** **Goal:** To assess respiratory status by evaluating rate and quality. **COMMENTS**
___	___	___	1. After assessment of pulse, keep fingers resting on client's wrist and observe or feel the rising and falling of chest with respiration. If client is asleep, gently place hand on client's chest to feel chest movement. *Do not* explain procedure to client.
___	___	___	2. When one complete cycle of inspiration and expiration has been observed, look at second hand of watch and count the number of complete cycles. If rate is regular in an adult, count 30 seconds and multiply by two. In children under 2 years of age or adults with irregular rate, count for one full minute.
___	___	___	3. If respirations are shallow and difficult to count, observe at the sternal notch.
___	___	___	4. Note depth and rhythm of respiratory cycle.
___	___	___	5. Discuss findings with client, if applicable.
___	___	___	6. Document respiratory rate, depth, rhythm, and character.

Procedure Checklists to Accompany Craven/Hirnle's Fundamentals of Nursing: Human Health and Function, third edition.

Name _____ Date _____

Unit _____ Position _____

Instructor/Evaluator _____ Position _____

Excellent ▼	Satisfactory ▼	Needs Practice ▼	

Procedure 23-4

Obtaining Blood Pressure

Goal: To evaluate the client's hemodynamic status by obtaining information about cardiac output, blood volume, peripheral vascular resistance, and arterial wall elasticity.

COMMENTS

1. Wash hands.
2. Explain procedure to client.
3. Assist client to comfortable position with forearm supported at heart level and palm up.
4. Expose upper arm completely.
5. Wrap deflated cuff snugly around upper arm with center of bladder over brachial artery. Lower border of cuff is 2 cm above antecubital space in an adult, and nearer the antecubital space in an infant.
6. If using mercury manometer, the manometer is vertical and at eye level.
7. Palpate brachial or radial artery with fingertips. Close valve on pressure bulb and inflate cuff until pulse disappears. Inflate 30 mmHg higher. Slowly release valve and note reading when pulse reappears.
8. Fully deflate cuff, and wait 1–2 minutes.
9. Place stethoscope ear pieces in ears. Repalpate the brachial artery and place stethoscope diaphragm or bell over site.
10. Close bulb valve by turning clockwise. Inflate cuff to 30 mmHg above reading at which brachial pulse disappeared.
11. Slowly release valve so pressure drops about 2–3 mmHg per second.
12. Identify manometer reading when first clear Korotkoff sound is heard.

Procedure 23-4

Obtaining Blood Pressure (continued)

Excellent ▼	Satisfactory ▼	Needs Practice ▼		COMMENTS
___	___	___	13. Continue to deflate, and note reading when sound muffles or dampens (fourth Korotkoff) and when it disappears (fifth Korotkoff).	
___	___	___	14. Deflate cuff completely and remove from client's arm.	
___	___	___	15. Record blood pressure. Record systolic and diastolic in the form 130/80. If three readings are to be recorded, use the form 130/80/40. Abbreviate RA or LA to indicate right or left arm measurement.	
___	___	___	16. Assist client to comfortable position, and discuss findings with client, if appropriate.	

Procedure Checklists to Accompany Craven/Hirnle's Fundamentals of Nursing: Human Health and Function, third edition.

Name _____ Date _____

Unit _____ Position _____

Instructor/Evaluator _____ Position _____

Excellent ▼	Satisfactory ▼	Needs Practice ▼	Procedure 23-5 **Assessing for Orthostatic Hypotension**	COMMENTS
			Goal: To assess the compensatory status of the cardiovascular and autonomic nervous systems to changes in body position.	
____	____	____	1. Wash hands. Explain procedure to client.	
____	____	____	2. Position client supine with head of bed flat for 10 minutes.	
____	____	____	3. Check and record supine blood pressure and pulse.	
____	____	____	4. Assist client to a sitting position with legs dangling over the edge of bed. Wait 2 minutes and check blood pressure and pulse rate.	
____	____	____	5. Assist client to standing position. Wait 2 minutes and check blood pressure and pulse rate. Be alert to signs and symptoms of dizziness.	
____	____	____	6. Assist client back to comfortable position.	
____	____	____	7. Record measurements and any symptoms that accompanied the postural change.	
____	____	____	8. Discuss findings with client, if appropriate.	

Procedure Checklists to Accompany Craven/Hirnle's Fundamentals of Nursing: Human Health and Function, third edition.

Name _____ Date _____

Unit _____ Position _____

Instructor/Evaluator _____ Position _____

Excellent	Satisfactory	Needs Practice	*Procedure 25-1* **Handwashing** **Goal:** To prevent transfer of microorganisms from health care personnel to client and from client to health care personnel.	COMMENTS
▼	▼	▼		
___	___	___	1. Remove all rings except a plain wedding band. Push watch 4–5 inches above wrist.	
___	___	___	2. Turn on the water and adjust temperature to warm. Do not splash water or lean against the wet sink.	
___	___	___	3. Hold hands lower than elbows and thoroughly wet hands and lower arms under running water.	
___	___	___	4. Apply soap and rub palms, wrists, and back of hands firmly with circular movements. Interlace fingers and thumbs, moving hands back and forth. Continue using plenty of lather and friction for 15–30 seconds on each hand. Timing of scrub may vary depending on purpose of wash and the amount of contamination.	
___	___	___	5. Clean under fingernails using fingernails of other hand and additional soap. Use orangewood stick, if available.	
___	___	___	6. Dry hands and arms thoroughly with paper towel, wiping from fingertips toward forearm. Discard in proper receptacle.	
___	___	___	7. Turn off water using clean, dry paper towel on faucets.	

Procedure Checklists to Accompany Craven/Hirnle's Fundamentals of Nursing: Human Health and Function, third edition.

Name _____ Date _____

Unit _____ Position _____

Instructor/Evaluator _____ Position _____

Excellent	Satisfactory	Needs Practice	
▼	▼	▼	*Procedure 25-2* # Donning and Removing a Mask and Gown **Goal:** To prevent spread of microorganisms from nurse to client, from client to nurse, and from nurse's clothing.

COMMENTS

Donning Mask

___	___	___	1. Wash hands.
___	___	___	2. If required, position mask over mouth and nose. Bend nose bar over bridge of nose. Secure strings or elastic.
___	___	___	3. Change mask if used for more than 30 minutes or when damp. Mask should never be allowed to hang around neck.

Donning Clean Gown

___	___	___	1. Grasp gown by collar allowing it to unfold. Place arms through sleeve and pull gown over shoulders.
___	___	___	2. Fasten neck ties. Overlap gown at back and fasten waist ties.

Removing Contaminated Gown

___	___	___	1. Untie waist ties and let gown hang freely.
___	___	___	2. Wash hands.
___	___	___	3. Untie neck ties and let gown fall forward off shoulders.
___	___	___	4. Slide arms out of gown, working from inside.
___	___	___	5. Holding gown away from your body, fold contaminated side of gown toward the inside.
___	___	___	6. Discard in appropriate receptacle.
___	___	___	7. Remove and discard mask.
___	___	___	8. Wash hands.

Procedure Checklists to Accompany Craven/Hirnle's Fundamentals of Nursing: Human Health and Function, third edition.

Name _____   Date _____

Unit _____   Position _____

Instructor/Evaluator _____   Position _____

Excellent	Satisfactory	Needs Practice	
▼	▼	▼	**Procedure 25-3** **Applying and Removing Sterile Gloves** **Goal:** To prevent transfer of microorganisms from hands to sterile objects or open wounds.

COMMENTS

Applying Gloves

___	___	___	1. Wash hands.
___	___	___	2. Remove outside wrapper by peeling apart sides.
___	___	___	3. Lay inner package on clean, flat surface above waist level. Open wrapper from the outside keeping gloves on inside surface.
___	___	___	4. Grasp inside edge of right cuff with thumb and first two fingers of dominant hand. Holding hands above waist, insert nondominant hand into glove. Adjust fingers inside glove after both gloves are on.
___	___	___	5. Slip gloved hand underneath second gloved cuff still in package, and pull over dominant hand.
___	___	___	6. Keeping hands above waist, adjust glove fit, touching only sterile areas.

Removing Gloves

___	___	___	1. With dominant hand, grasp outer surface of nondominant glove just below thumb. Peel off without touching exposed wrist.
___	___	___	2. Place ungloved hand under thumb side of second cuff and peel off toward fingers, holding first glove inside second glove. Discard into appropriate receptacle.
___	___	___	3. Wash hands.

Procedure Checklists to Accompany Craven/Hirnle's Fundamentals of Nursing: Human Health and Function, third edition.

Name _____ Date _____

Unit _____ Position _____

Instructor/Evaluator _____ Position _____

Excellent ▼	Satisfactory ▼	Needs Practice ▼		COMMENTS
			Procedure 26-1 **Administering Oral Medications** **Goal:** To provide a safe, effective, economic route for administering medications.	
____	____	____	1. Wash hands.	
____	____	____	2. Arrange Medication Administration Record (MAR) next to medication cart or cabinet, medication trays, and cups.	
____	____	____	3. Prepare medications for only one client at a time.	
____	____	____	4. Remove ordered medications from cart or shelf. Compare label on medication with MAR and check the five rights of medication administration. If a discrepancy exists, recheck the client's chart and medication orders.	
____	____	____	5. Calculate correct drug dosage, if necessary.	
____	____	____	6. Compare medications with MAR and recheck the five rights of medication administration.	
____	____	____	7. Prepare selected medications.	
____	____	____	a. Unit dosage: Place packaged medications directly into medicine cup, or lay on tray without unwrapping.	
____	____	____	b. Medications from a multidose bottle: Pour tablets or capsules into the container lid, and transfer into medicine cup. Return any extra tablets to the bottle.	
____	____	____	c. Medications from a bingo card: Snap the bubble containing the correct medication directly over the medicine cup. Do not touch medications.	
____	____	____	d. Swallowing difficulty: If client has trouble swallowing tablets, grind with mortar and pestle or other drug-crushing device until smooth. Mix powder in small amount of pudding or applesauce. Do not crush enteric-coated tablets or extended-release tablets.	

Procedure 26-1

Administering Oral Medications (continued)

Excellent	Satisfactory	Needs Practice		COMMENTS
▼	▼	▼		
___	___	___	e. Liquid medications: Remove cap and place on counter-top inside up. Hold bottle so label is against palm of hand. Hold medication cup at eye level, and fill until bottom of meniscus is at desired dosage. Discard excess poured liquid from cup into sink. Do not pour back into bottle.	
___	___	___	8. Take medication directly to client's room. Do not leave medication unattended.	
___	___	___	9. Compare name on MAR with name on client's identification band. If the client is not wearing an identification band, ask the client to state his or her name.	
___	___	___	10. Complete any preadministration assessment.	
___	___	___	11. Compare medication to MAR, and recheck the five rights of medication administration. If using unit dose medications, unwrap the medication and place in the cup before checking the five rights of the next medication.	
___	___	___	12. Explain medication's purpose to client.	
___	___	___	13. Assist client to sitting position, if necessary. Give medication cup and glass of water to client.	
___	___	___	14. If client is unable to hold the medication cup, place pill cup to lips and introduce medication into his or her mouth. If tablet or capsule falls on floor, discard and repeat preparation.	
___	___	___	15. Stay with client until he or she swallows all medications. Look inside client's mouth if the client is cognitively impaired or has difficulty swallowing to ensure client receives the ordered medications.	
___	___	___	16. Dispose of soiled supplies and wash hands.	
___	___	___	17. Document the time that medication was administered and any preadministration assessment data collected.	

26

Procedure Checklists to Accompany Craven/Hirnle's Fundamentals of Nursing: Human Health and Function, third edition.

Name _____ Date _____

Unit _____ Position _____

Instructor/Evaluator _____ Position _____

Procedure 26-2
Administering Medication by Metered-Dose Inhaler (MDI)

Goal: To deliver premeasured dose of medication to the bronchial airways and lungs.

Columns: Excellent ▼ | Satisfactory ▼ | Needs Practice ▼

COMMENTS

1. Check medication order.
2. Compare the medication with the MAR, and recheck the five rights of medication administration.
3. Wash hands.
4. Assemble medication canister, inhalation mouthpiece, and spacer device, if needed. Attach the medication canister to the inhaler mouthpiece by inserting the metal stem into the long end of the mouthpiece. Shake the canister several times.
5. Assist the client to sitting or standing position. Perform the third medication check.
6. Ask client to breathe out through his or her mouth.
7. Position the mouthpiece 1–2 inches from client's open mouth. Instruct the client to breathe in slowly through his or her mouth. As client starts inhaling, press the canister down to release one dose of the medication.
8. Instruct client to hold his or her breath for 10 seconds, if possible.
9. Wait at least one minute before administration of a second dose or inhalation of a different medication by MDI. Administer bronchodilators by MDI before other inhaled medications.
10. Wash hands and clean mouthpiece. If steroid medication was administered, have client rinse mouth.
11. Reassess ease of breathing, respiratory rate, accessory muscle use, and breath sounds.

Copyright © 2000 by Lippincott Williams & Wilkins. Procedure Checklists to Accompany Craven/Hirnle's *Fundamentals of Nursing: Human Health and Function,* third edition by Elissa Swisher Sauer

Procedure 26-2

Administering Medication by Metered-Dose Inhaler (MDI) (continued)

Excellent	Satisfactory	Needs Practice		COMMENTS
___	___	___	12. Document medication administration and client status before and after administration.	

Modification for Using a Spacer with an MDI

___	___	___	13. Attach spacer to inhalation mouthpiece. After exhaling, instruct client to place the mouthpiece in his or her mouth and close lips around the mouthpiece. Depress the medication canister and have client inhale. If client can't take or hold a deep breath, advise to take two or three short breaths to get all the medication from the spacer.	

Procedure Checklists to Accompany Craven/Hirnle's Fundamentals of Nursing: Human Health and Function, third edition.

Name _____   Date _____

Unit _____   Position _____

Instructor/Evaluator _____   Position _____

Excellent ▼	Satisfactory ▼	Needs Practice ▼	*Procedure 26-3* **Withdrawing Medication from a Vial** **Goal:** To withdraw a precise amount of medication from a vial without introducing contamination.	COMMENTS
___	___	___	1. Check medication order and compare the name of the ordered medication with the label on the medication vial. Follow Steps 1–6 of Procedure 26-1.	
___	___	___	2. Assemble needle and syringe.	
___	___	___	3. Pick up vial. If medication has been reconstituted or is in suspension, place vial between the palms, rotating or rolling the vial back and forth.	
___	___	___	4. Remove metal cap from vial.	
___	___	___	5. Cleanse top of vial with alcohol wipe.	
___	___	___	6. Remove guard from needle.	
___	___	___	7. Pull back on barrel of syringe to draw in a volume of air equal to the volume of the ordered medication dose.	
___	___	___	8. Holding vial between thumb and fingers of the nondominant hand, insert needle through the rubber stopper into the air space—not the solution—in the vial and inject air.	
___	___	___	9. Invert vial and withdraw the ordered dose of medication by pulling back on the plunger. Make sure needle is in the solution to be withdrawn.	
___	___	___	10. Expel air bubbles and adjust dose, if necessary.	
___	___	___	11. Remove needle from vial and cover the needle with guard.	
___	___	___	12. Wash hands.	

Name _____ Date _____

Unit _____ Position _____

Instructor/Evaluator _____ Position _____

Procedure 26-4

Withdrawing Medication from an Ampule

Goal: To withdraw full dose of medication from an ampule safely and without introducing contamination.

Columns: Excellent ▼ | Satisfactory ▼ | Needs Practice ▼ — COMMENTS

1. Check medication order and make sure the solution in the ampule matches the ordered solution.
2. Complete Steps 1–6 of Procedure 26-1.
3. Assemble needle and syringe.
4. Pick up ampule and flick its upper stem several times with a fingernail.
5. Wrap a sterile gauze pad or alcohol wipe around the neck of the ampule before breaking the neck with an outward, snapping motion.
6. Discard the broken neck appropriately, and prepare to withdraw medication from ampule using one of two methods:
   a. Place ampule upright on a flat surface, insert needle in the solution, and withdraw the correct amount of medication by pulling up on the plunger without touching the needle to the glass rim.
   b. Alternatively, invert the ampule or tilt it sideways. Insert the needle into the solution, pull back on the plunger, and withdraw the proper dose of medication.
7. Remove needle from solution. Hold needle upright, inspect the syringe, and dispel any air that may have been drawn into the syringe. Make sure the syringe contains the correct amount of medication. Expel any extra medication into a container.
8. Cover needle with guard and discard ampule in sharps container.
9. Wash hands.

Procedure Checklists to Accompany Craven/Hirnle's Fundamentals of Nursing: Human Health and Function, third edition.

Name _____ Date _____

Unit _____ Position _____

Instructor/Evaluator _____ Position _____

Excellent ▼	Satisfactory ▼	Needs Practice ▼	*Procedure 26-5* **Drawing Up Two Medications in a Syringe** **Goal:** To minimize the number of injections a client receives and to prevent contamination of one medication vial with medication from another.	COMMENTS
___	___	___	1. Wash hands.	
___	___	___	2. Compare medications to MAR. Complete Steps 1–6 of Procedure 26-1.	
___	___	___	3. Cleanse tops of both vials with antiseptic.	
___	___	___	4. With syringe, aspirate volume of air equal to medication dose from first medication (Vial A).	
___	___	___	5. Inject air into Vial A, being careful that needle does not touch solution.	
___	___	___	6. Remove syringe from Vial A. Aspirate volume of air equal to the medication dose from second medication (Vial B). Inject air into Vial B.	
___	___	___	7. Invert Vial B, and withdraw required volume of medication into syringe. Expel all air bubbles and withdraw needle from Vial B.	
___	___	___	8. Determine what total combined volume of medication would measure on syringe scale.	
___	___	___	9. Insert needle into Vial A, invert vial, and carefully withdraw required volume of medication.	
___	___	___	10. Withdraw needle from Vial A and replace needle guard.	
___	___	___	11. Check medication and dosage before returning or discarding vials.	

Procedure 26-5

Drawing Up Two Medications in a Syringe (continued)

Excellent	Satisfactory	Needs Practice		COMMENTS
▼	▼	▼		

Modification for Insulin

___	___	___	1. Wash hands.
___	___	___	2. When preparing insulin in suspension, gently rotate vials between palms of hands to mix the suspension.
___	___	___	3. Repeat Steps 3–9.
___	___	___	4. Draw regular insulin into the syringe first.

Procedure Checklists to Accompany Craven/Hirnle's Fundamentals of Nursing: Human Health and Function, third edition.

Name _____ Date _____

Unit _____ Position _____

Instructor/Evaluator _____ Position _____

Excellent	Satisfactory	Needs Practice		COMMENTS
▼	▼	▼	**Procedure 26-6** **Administering an Intradermal Injection** **Goal:** To administer medication into dermal tissue to screen for allergic dermal reactions.	
____	____	____	1. Check medication order. Follow Steps 1–5 of Procedure 26-1.	
____	____	____	2. Assemble needle and syringe.	
____	____	____	3. Recheck five rights against MAR.	
____	____	____	4. Remove needle guard and withdraw medication from vial.	
____	____	____	5. Identify client by name or identification bracelet. Explain procedure to client.	
____	____	____	6. Perform third check of five rights.	
____	____	____	7. Select injection site that is relatively hairless and free from tenderness, swelling, scarring, or inflammation.	
____	____	____	8. Remove needle guard. Hold syringe in dominant hand. Gently pull skin distal to intended injection site taut with nondominant hand.	
____	____	____	9. Holding syringe from above, at a 10- to 15-degree angle (almost parallel to skin), gently insert needle, bevel up, until dermis barely covers bevel.	
____	____	____	10. Stabilize needle, then inject medication slowly over 3–5 seconds.	
____	____	____	11. Withdraw needle. Do *not* wipe or massage site.	
____	____	____	12. Do not recap needle. Dispose of syringe and needle in sharps container.	
____	____	____	13. Record time and site of injection according to agency protocol.	
____	____	____	14. Instruct client when to return for reading of response—15–60 minutes after injection for allergy testing, usually 48–72 hours after injection for Tuberculin skin testing (TST).	

Procedure Checklists to Accompany Craven/Hirnle's Fundamentals of Nursing: Human Health and Function, third edition.

Name _____ Date _____

Unit _____ Position _____

Instructor/Evaluator _____ Position _____

Excellent ▼	Satisfactory ▼	Needs Practice ▼	
			Procedure 26-7

Administering Subcutaneous Injections

Goal: To ensure more rapid absorption and action of a medication than can be achieved orally.

COMMENTS

Excellent	Satisfactory	Needs Practice	
___	___	___	1. Check medication order. Follow Steps 1–5 of Procedure 26-1.
___	___	___	2. Assemble needle and syringe.
___	___	___	3. Recheck five rights against MAR.
___	___	___	4. Remove needle guard and withdraw medication from container (see Procedures 26-3 and 26-4).
___	___	___	5. Identify client by name or identification bracelet. Explain procedure to client.
___	___	___	6. Perform third check of five rights.
___	___	___	7. Don gloves.
___	___	___	8. Select injection site that is free from tenderness, swelling, scarring, and inflammation.
___	___	___	9. Cleanse site with antiseptic swab in circular motion from center outward. Allow area to dry thoroughly.
___	___	___	10. Remove needle guard. Hold syringe in dominant hand. Place nondominant hand on either side of injection site. Spread or bunch skin to stabilize site and identify subcutaneous tissue.
___	___	___	11. Hold syringe between thumb and forefinger of dominant hand. Inject needle quickly at a 45- to 90-degree angle.
___	___	___	12. Aspirate by slowly pulling back on plunger. If blood appears in syringe, withdraw needle, discard syringe, and prepare a new injection.
___	___	___	13. If no blood appears, inject medication with slow, even pressure.
___	___	___	14. Remove needle quickly while pressing antiseptic swab over site.

Procedure 26-7

Administering Subcutaneous Injections (continued)

Excellent	Satisfactory	Needs Practice		COMMENTS
▼	▼	▼		
⎯	⎯	⎯	15. Gently massage site with antiseptic swab.	
⎯	⎯	⎯	16. Do not recap needle. Dispose of syringe and needle in sharps container.	
⎯	⎯	⎯	17. Wash hands.	
⎯	⎯	⎯	18. Record according to agency protocol.	
			Modification for Insulin Administration	
⎯	⎯	⎯	1. Routine aspiration is not necessary.	
⎯	⎯	⎯	2. Systematically rotate injection sites to prevent lipodystrophy and variable insulin absorption.	
⎯	⎯	⎯	3. Instruct clients who self-administer insulin about not needing to cleanse site with alcohol or to wear gloves.	
			Modification for Heparin Administration	
⎯	⎯	⎯	1. The abdomen, except for 1–2 inches on either side of umbilicus, is the most frequently used site.	
⎯	⎯	⎯	2. Roll or gently bunch tissue between thumb and forefinger to ensure heparin is administered into subcutaneous tissue. Do not pinch skin tightly.	
⎯	⎯	⎯	3. Do not aspirate for blood return or massage skin after injection.	
⎯	⎯	⎯	4. After injection, slowly and smoothly withdraw needle to prevent leakage into subcutaneous tissue.	

Procedure Checklists to Accompany Craven/Hirnle's Fundamentals of Nursing: Human Health and Function, third edition.

Name _____ Date _____

Unit _____ Position _____

Instructor/Evaluator _____ Position _____

Excellent ▼	Satisfactory ▼	Needs Practice ▼	*Procedure 26-8* **Administering Intramuscular Injections** **Goal:** To administer medication deeply into muscle tissue, without injury to client.	COMMENTS
____	____	____	1. Check medication order. See Procedure 26-1, Steps 1–5. Assemble needle and syringe.	
____	____	____	2. Recheck five rights of medication against MAR.	
____	____	____	3. Prepare needle, syringe, and medication by following appropriate steps in Procedure 26-3 or Procedure 26-4.	
____	____	____	4. If medication is known to be irritating to subcutaneous tissues, replace needle after withdrawing medication.	
____	____	____	5. Identify client by name or identification bracelet. Explain procedure to client.	
____	____	____	6. Don gloves. Assist client to a comfortable position, and expose only the area to be injected.	
____	____	____	7. Select appropriate injection site by inspecting muscle size and integrity. Consider volume of medication to be injected.	
____	____	____	8. Use anatomic landmarks to locate exact injection site.	
____	____	____	9. Cleanse site with antiseptic swab, wiping from center of site and rotating outward.	
____	____	____	10. Remove needle guard. Hold syringe between thumb and forefinger of dominant hand (like a dart). Spread skin at the site with nondominant hand.	
____	____	____	11. Insert needle quickly at a 90-degree angle to client's skin surface.	
____	____	____	12. Stabilize syringe barrel by grasping with nondominant hand:	
____	____	____	a. Aspirate slowly by pulling back on plunger with dominant hand.	

Procedure 26-8
Administering Intramuscular Injections (continued)

Excellent	Satisfactory	Needs Practice		COMMENTS
▼	▼	▼		
—	—	—	b. If no blood appears, inject medication slowly.	
—	—	—	c. If blood appears in syringe, remove needle, dispose of syringe, and prepare new medication.	
—	—	—	13. Withdraw needle while pressing antiseptic swab above site.	
—	—	—	14. Gently massage site.	
—	—	—	15. Do not recap needle. Dispose of equipment in sharps container.	
—	—	—	16. Wash hands.	
—	—	—	17. Record medication and client response according to agency protocol.	

Variation for Air-Lock Injection Technique

Excellent	Satisfactory	Needs Practice		
—	—	—	1. Withdraw desired volume of medication into syringe.	
—	—	—	2. Draw in an additional 0.2 mL of air.	
—	—	—	3. Check medication dose in syringe; expel excess amount of medication from syringe.	
—	—	—	4. Redraw in 0.2 mL of air, and recheck dose accuracy.	
—	—	—	5. Insert the needle entering the client at a 90-degree angle to the client's skin surface and the floor. Position the client so the proper anatomic landmarks can be located for the chosen site and still allow the needle to enter the client at a 90-degree angle to the floor.	

Variation for Z-Track Injection

Excellent	Satisfactory	Needs Practice		
—	—	—	1. When preparing injection site, pull skin and subcutaneous tissues about 1–1.5 inches to one side of the selected site.	
—	—	—	2. Insert syringe at a 90-degree angle.	
—	—	—	3. Aspirate and administer medication while continuing traction on skin.	
—	—	—	4. Leave needle inserted an additional 10 seconds.	
—	—	—	5. Simultaneously remove needle and release traction on skin.	

Procedure Checklists to Accompany Craven/Hirnle's Fundamentals of Nursing: Human Health and Function, third edition.

Name _____ Date _____

Unit _____ Position _____

Instructor/Evaluator _____ Position _____

Excellent	Satisfactory	Needs Practice	*Procedure 26-9* **Administering Medications by Intravenous Push** **Goal:** To achieve high blood levels of a medication in a short time period.	COMMENTS
▼	▼	▼		
___	___	___	1. Check medication order. See Procedure 26-1, Steps 1–5.	
___	___	___	2. Recheck the five rights of medication administration.	
___	___	___	3. Prepare and draw up ordered medication from vial or ampule. Read package insert for proper amount and solution for dilution. Apply needleless adaptor or a small-gauge needle to syringe.	
___	___	___	4. Identify client by looking at name band or by asking name. Perform the third check of the five rights.	
___	___	___	5. Explain procedure to client.	
___	___	___	6. Don gloves.	
			Administering Medication into an Existing IV Line	
___	___	___	1. Select injection port in IV tubing, closest to IV insertion site.	
___	___	___	2. If using a needle, cleanse injection port with antiseptic. Allow to dry.	
___	___	___	3. Insert needle into injection port or attach syringe to injection port (needleless system).	
___	___	___	4. Occlude the IV tubing above the injection port by pinching the tubing. Gently pull back on the syringe plunger until blood appears in the tubing.	
___	___	___	5. Inject medication slowly into the IV port at the prescribed rate. Use a watch to time administration rate.	
___	___	___	6. If IV medication and IV solution in tubing are incompatible, assess for blood return with 10-mL syringe of sterile normal saline solution.	

Excellent	Satisfactory	Needs Practice	

Procedure 26-9

Administering Medications by Intravenous Push (continued)

COMMENTS

—— —— —— 7. After confirming IV catheter placement, flush line with normal saline solution while occluding catheter above port.

—— —— —— 8. Administer medication at prescribed rate; reflush with 10 mL of sterile normal saline solution, and release occlusion.

Administering Medication into Intermittent Injection Device or Lock Device

—— —— —— 1. Swab the injection port with antiseptic. Allow to dry.

—— —— —— 2. Attach syringe (needleless system) or insert needle of syringe with one mL normal saline solution into injection port. Gently pull back on syringe plunger to assess for blood return.

—— —— —— 3. Flush IV lock with one mL normal saline solution. Remove syringe.

—— —— —— 4. Attach syringe (needleless system) or insert needle of syringe with medication into injection port. Inject medication slowly at the prescribed rate. Use watch to time safe administration rate. Remove syringe.

—— —— —— 5. Attach syringe (needleless system) or insert needle of syringe with 1–3 mL of normal saline into injection port and flush the port with saline.

—— —— —— 6. Dispose of uncapped needles and syringes in sharps container.

—— —— —— 7. Wash hands.

—— —— —— 8. Document medication administration.

—— —— —— 9. Evaluate client's response to medication therapy.

Procedure Checklists to Accompany Craven/Hirnle's Fundamentals of Nursing: Human Health and Function, third edition.

Name _____ Date _____

Unit _____ Position _____

Instructor/Evaluator _____ Position _____

Procedure 26-10

Administering IV Medications Using Intermittent Infusion Technique

Goal: To maintain therapeutic levels of medication in client's blood.

Excellent	Satisfactory	Needs Practice		COMMENTS
____	____	____	1. Check medication order. See Procedure 26-1, Steps 1–5.	
____	____	____	2. Recheck five rights of medication administration.	
____	____	____	3. Prepare the medication syringe and IV tubing. Examine the syringe for any air bubbles and expel any that are present. Attach the syringe to the extension tubing, and gently push the syringe plunger to prime tubing. Cover adaptor.	
____	____	____	4. Secure the medication syringe into the pump with the flange of the syringe in the clamp's groove.	
____	____	____	5. Confirm client's identity by looking at identification band or by asking his or her name. Perform the third check of the five rights and explain the procedure to the client.	
____	____	____	6. Don gloves.	
____	____	____	7. Cleanse injection port with alcohol swab and allow to dry.	
____	____	____	8. Attach syringe (needleless system) or insert needle of syringe with normal saline into the lock device. Flush lock with normal saline. Gently pull back on syringe plunger to assess for blood return.	
____	____	____	9. Attach tubing (needleless system) or tubing with needle to lock device. Secure IV tubing to IV site with tape.	
____	____	____	10. Program the pump for the appropriate infusion speed and press the "Start" key. The medication syringe label often indicates the suggested infusion speed, typically 30–60 minutes. If uncertain, consult a drug reference handbook or pharmacist.	
____	____	____	11. Document medication administration.	

Administering IV Medications Using Intermittent Infusion Technique (continued)

Excellent ▼	Satisfactory ▼	Needs Practice ▼		COMMENTS
――	――	――	12. Assess client and infusion device 5–10 minutes after infusion has begun.	
――	――	――	13. When the completion alarm sounds, return to client's room and press the pump's "Stop" key.	
――	――	――	14. Don gloves. Remove tubing from lock device. Attach syringe (needleless system) or insert needle of second syringe with 1–3 mL normal saline or heparin flush solution and flush lock.	
――	――	――	15. Replace lock with new sterile cap (needleless system).	
――	――	――	16. Dispose of uncapped needles and syringes in sharps container.	
――	――	――	17. Wash hands.	
			Variation Using IV Bag and Gravity IV Tubing	
――	――	――	1. Follow Steps 1 and 2 above.	
――	――	――	2. Connect infusion tubing to medication bag (see Procedure 27-2).	
――	――	――	3. Follow Steps 6–9 above.	
――	――	――	4. Set IV drip rate to infuse medication over prescribed time. Monitor periodically.	
――	――	――	5. Document medication administration.	
――	――	――	6. When medication has infused, turn off flow clamp.	
――	――	――	7. Follow Steps 14–17 above.	
			Variation When Administering Intermittent IV Medication into Primary IV Line	
――	――	――	1. Perform previous steps through second check of five rights.	
――	――	――	2. Prepare medication, tubing, and pump, if used according to procedures described above.	
――	――	――	3. Confirm client's identity and perform third medication check.	

Procedure 26-10

Administering IV Medications Using Intermittent Infusion Technique (continued)

COMMENTS

Excellent	Satisfactory	Needs Practice	
▼	▼	▼	
___	___	___	4. Hang syringe pump or medication bag at or above level of primary IV solution.
___	___	___	a. If using a needle, wipe injection port nearest IV insertion site on primary IV tubing with antiseptic and attach needle with needle protector.
___	___	___	b. If using a needleless system, insert secondary line into the needleless adaptor port.
___	___	___	5. Check compatibility of medications to be administered with the IV solution being infused and any other infusing medications. If medications are not compatible with primary IV solution, clamp primary IV tubing above injection port, insert needle with 20-mL syringe of normal saline flush solution, and flush IV line.
___	___	___	6. Secure secondary tubing to primary tubing with tape.
___	___	___	7. Start syringe pump or set drip rate.
___	___	___	8. When medication has infused, stop syringe pump or turn off flow clamp. Flush IV line with saline, p.r.n. Regulate primary infusion as necessary.
___	___	___	9. Discard medication syringe or bag, tubing, and needle or needleless adaptor, or leave hanging with needle covered for future use, as dictated by agency policy.
___	___	___	10. Wash hands.
___	___	___	11. Document medication administration and add IV volume to IV intake.

Procedure Checklists to Accompany Craven/Hirnle's Fundamentals of Nursing: Human Health and Function, third edition.

Name _____ Date _____

Unit _____ Position _____

Instructor/Evaluator _____ Position _____

Excellent	Satisfactory	Needs Practice	
▼	▼	▼	**Procedure 27-1** **Monitoring an Intravenous Infusion** **Goal:** To provide a safe, patent route for infusion of IV fluid therapy.

COMMENTS

___	___	___	1. Compare IV fluid currently infusing with the ordered solution.
___	___	___	2. Inspect the rate of flow at least every hour. For other IVs, check actual flow rate for 15 seconds and compare with prescribed rate of flow. If infusion is ahead of schedule, slow it so the infusion will complete at the planned time. If infusion is behind schedule, review agency policy before increasing flow rate.
___	___	___	3. Inspect the system for leakage, and, if present, locate the source. Tighten all connections within the system. If leak is still present, slow IV flow rate to keep vein open and replace tubing with sterile set.
___	___	___	4. Inspect the tubing for kinks or blockages. Loosely coil tubing and place it on the bed.
___	___	___	5. Observe the fluid level in the drip chamber. If it is less than half-full, squeeze the chamber gently to allow more fluid in.
___	___	___	6. Inspect the infusion site for infiltration. Look for signs of infiltration, including decreased rate of flow, swelling, pallor, coolness, and discomfort at or above the needle insertion site. If present, change the IV site. If a large amount of fluid infiltrated, elevate the client's arm above the heart on several pillows.
___	___	___	7. Inspect client's arm above the insertion point for signs of phlebitis, including redness, swelling, warmth, and pain along the vein above the IV insertion site. If present, discontinue the IV and restart in another area.
___	___	___	8. Inspect the insertion site for bleeding.

Excellent	Satisfactory	Needs Practice	Procedure 27-1 **Monitoring an Intravenous Infusion (continued)**	COMMENTS
___	___	___	9. If able to comply, teach client to contact the nurse if any of the following occur: • The flow rate changes suddenly. • The fluid container is almost empty. • Blood is in the tubing. • The site becomes uncomfortable.	
___	___	___	10. Document any findings indicating complications of IV therapy (e.g., infiltration).	

44

Procedure Checklists to Accompany Craven/Hirnle's Fundamentals of Nursing: Human Health and Function, third edition.

Name _____ Date _____

Unit _____ Position _____

Instructor/Evaluator _____ Position _____

Excellent ▼	Satisfactory ▼	Needs Practice ▼	*Procedure 27-2* **Changing Intravenous Solution and Tubing**	COMMENTS
			Goal: To deliver IV therapy as ordered and decrease risk of client infection.	
			Changing Solution Container	
——	——	——	1. Wash hands and explain procedure to client.	
——	——	——	2. Compare solution with physician's order. Adhere to five rights of medication administration.	
——	——	——	3. Remove IV bag from outer wrapper.	
——	——	——	4. Label solution container with client's name, solution type, additives, date, and time hung. Check prelabeled container with physician's order. Line up time strip with volume amount on bag or bottle. Record solution change in the client's record.	
——	——	——	5. Prepare container for spiking:	
——	——	——	a. If solution is in a plastic bag, remove plastic cover from entry nipple. Maintain sterility of nipple end.	
——	——	——	b. If solution is in a bottle, remove metal cap, metal disk, and rubber disk. Maintain sterility of bottle top.	
——	——	——	6. Close clamp on the existing tubing.	
——	——	——	7. Take old solution container from pole and invert it.	
——	——	——	8. Remove spike from used container, maintaining its sterility. Spike new IV container with firm push/twist motion.	
——	——	——	9. Hang new container on IV pole.	
——	——	——	10. Inspect tubing for air bubbles, and assess that drip chamber is one-half full of solution.	
——	——	——	11. Adjust clamp to regulate flow rate, according to orders.	

Copyright © 2000 by Lippincott Williams & Wilkins. Procedure Checklists to Accompany Craven/Hirnle's *Fundamentals of Nursing: Human Health and Function,* third edition by Elissa Swisher Sauer

Procedure 27-2

Changing Intravenous Solution and Tubing (continued)

Excellent	Satisfactory	Needs Practice		COMMENTS
▼	▼	▼		

Changing Solution and Tubing

___	___	___	1. Follow first three steps of above procedure.
___	___	___	2. Open new tubing package, keeping protective covers on spike and catheter adapter.
___	___	___	3. Adjust roller clamp on new tubing to fully closed position.
___	___	___	4. Prepare new solution container as directed in Step 5 above.
___	___	___	5. Remove protective cover from spike, maintaining sterility, and spike into new solution container.
___	___	___	6. Hang container and "prime" drip chamber by squeezing gently, allowing to fill one-half full.
___	___	___	7. Remove protective cap from catheter adapter and adjust roller clamp to flush tubing with fluid. Replace protective cap.
___	___	___	8. Adjust roller clamp on old tubing to close fully.
___	___	___	9. Place towel or disposable underpad under extremity. Don clean, disposable gloves.
___	___	___	10. Hold catheter hub with fingers of one hand. With other hand, loosen tubing using gentle twisting motion. Remove old dressings, if necessary.
___	___	___	11. Grasp new tubing, remove protective catheter cap, and insert tightly into needle hub, while continuing to stabilize catheter hub with the other hand.
___	___	___	12. Adjust roller clamp to start solution flowing, according to physician's order.
___	___	___	13. Remove and discard gloves.
___	___	___	14. Secure tubing with tape.
___	___	___	15. If dressing was removed, apply new dressing to IV site according to agency policy.
___	___	___	16. Label new tubing with date, time, and your initials.
___	___	___	17. Label solution container with client's name, solution type, additives, date, and time hung. Time label side of container.
___	___	___	18. Document change of solution and tubing on client's record.

Procedure Checklists to Accompany Craven/Hirnle's Fundamentals of Nursing: Human Health and Function, third edition.

Name _____ Date _____

Unit _____ Position _____

Instructor/Evaluator _____ Position _____

Procedure 27-3

Converting to an Intermittent Infusion Device (IID) and Flushing

Goal: To maintain patency of intermittently used intravenous lock.

Excellent	Satisfactory	Needs Practice		COMMENTS
▼	▼	▼		
___	___	___	1. Wash hands.	
___	___	___	2. Explain procedure to client.	
___	___	___	3. Prepare syringe with heparin flush solution or saline solution according to agency policy and manufacturer's recommendations for the type of device in place (may use between 0.5–1 mL [peripheral], 2.5–3 mL [central line] heparin flush, or 1–3 mL normal saline).	
___	___	___	4. Obtain appropriate IID.	
___	___	___	5. Don clean gloves.	
			Converting IV to an Intermittent Infusion Device (IID)	
___	___	___	1. Clamp tubing of IV infusion with roller clamp.	
___	___	___	2. Hold the catheter hub firmly with your nondominant hand. With dominant hand, quickly twist IV tubing to the left to loosen but not disconnect from IV catheter.	
___	___	___	3. Take IID out of package, keeping tip sterile. Hold in dominant hand between thumb and finger.	
___	___	___	4. Stabilize IV catheter with nondominant hand as you disconnect IV tubing. Quickly insert IID into IV catheter, twisting to the right to tighten.	
___	___	___	5. Tape IID to stabilize. Redress using transparent dressing, if necessary.	
			Flushing with Needle Type System	
___	___	___	1. Perform Steps 1–5 above.	
___	___	___	2. Swab injection port with antiseptic swab and allow to dry.	

Excellent	Satisfactory	Needs Practice		

Procedure 27-3

Converting to an Intermittent Infusion Device (IID) and Flushing (continued)

COMMENTS

___ ___ ___   3. Insert needle into the port and aspirate gently for evidence of blood return.

___ ___ ___   4. Inject the recommended amount of saline or heparin flush, ending with 0.5 mL of solution remaining in syringe.

___ ___ ___   5. Dispose of uncapped needles and syringes in sharps container.

___ ___ ___   6. Wash hands.

___ ___ ___   7. Document date, time, route, amount, and type of flush solution. Also document assessment of site.

Flushing with Needleless System

   1. Perform Steps 1–5 above.

___ ___ ___   2. Remove protective wrapper from device.

___ ___ ___   3. Attach syringe, with needle removed, to intravenous catheter.

___ ___ ___   4. Aspirate gently, observing for blood return in the catheter.

___ ___ ___   5. Slowly inject the saline or heparin flush into the catheter ending with 0.5 mL of solution in syringe.

___ ___ ___   6. Remove syringe from catheter and cap end with a new sterile end protector.

___ ___ ___   7. Wash hands.

___ ___ ___   8. Document date, time, route, amount, and type of flush solution. Also document assessment of site.

Procedure Checklists to Accompany Craven/Hirnle's Fundamentals of Nursing: Human Health and Function, third edition.

Name _____ Date _____

Unit _____ Position _____

Instructor/Evaluator _____ Position _____

Procedure 27-4

Administering Total Parenteral Nutrition (TPN)

Goal: To provide parenteral nutritional support to selected clients.

Excellent	Satisfactory	Needs Practice		COMMENTS
▼	▼	▼		
			Monitoring TPN Therapy	
——	——	——	1. Schedule and assist client with chest x-ray after central catheter insertion.	
——	——	——	2. Confirm correct solution is running at ordered rate. Check expiration date of solution. Use infusion controller to monitor and regulate flow rate. Infuse solutions with 10% dextrose or more directly into subclavian or internal jugular vein to rapidly dilute the solution and prevent thrombophlebitis.	
——	——	——	3. Inspect tubing and catheter connection for leaks or kinks. Tape all connections. Change tubing every 24 hours according to agency policy.	
——	——	——	4. Inspect insertion site for infiltration, thrombophlebitis, or drainage. If present, notify physician.	
——	——	——	5. Monitor vital signs, including temperature, every 4 hours.	
——	——	——	6. Assess for symptoms of air embolism, i.e., decreased level of consciousness, tachycardia, dyspnea, anxiety, "feeling of impending doom," chest pain, cyanosis, hypotension. If suspected, lay patient on left side with head in Trendelenburg position.	
——	——	——	7. Use TPN line *only* for TPN.	
——	——	——	8. Perform test for glucose every 6 hours. Notify physician if abnormal.	
——	——	——	9. Monitor laboratory tests of electrolytes, BUN, glucose, as ordered, and report abnormal findings.	

Procedure 27-4

Administering Total Parenteral Nutrition (TPN) (continued)

Excellent	Satisfactory	Needs Practice		COMMENTS
▼	▼	▼		
___	___	___	10. Maintain accurate record of intake and output to monitor fluid balance.	
___	___	___	11. Weigh client daily and record.	
___	___	___	12. Inspect dressing once per shift for drainage and intactness. Change whenever loose or moist, and at least every 48 hours.	

Changing TPN Tubing and Dressing

___	___	___	1. Wash hands.	
___	___	___	2. Cross-check new hyperalimentation solutions with physician's order. Check expiration date.	
___	___	___	3. Attach sterile tubing and filter to new parenteral hyperalimentation solutions.	
___	___	___	4. Prime tubing as for a conventional IV.	
___	___	___	5. Place client in supine position.	
___	___	___	6. Don a mask. Instruct client to turn head facing opposite direction of insertion site, and not to cough or talk during dressing change. (Place mask on client if unable to cooperate.)	
___	___	___	7. Don gloves.	
___	___	___	8. Remove old dressing and discard carefully.	
___	___	___	9. Inspect insertion site for redness, drainage, or swelling.	
___	___	___	10. Remove gloves.	
___	___	___	11. Wash hands.	
___	___	___	12. Open sterile supplies and place on bedside table.	
___	___	___	13. Put on sterile gloves.	
___	___	___	14. Cleanse insertion site with gauze soaked in 10% acetone. Wipe in circular motion, moving from the insertion site outward without touching catheter with acetone.	
___	___	___	15. Cleanse site with same circular motion for 2 minutes using povidone-iodine solution (Betadine). Allow to air dry.	
___	___	___	16. Cleanse connection of catheter and tubing with Betadine.	
___	___	___	17. Remove Betadine from skin with alcohol, according to agency policy.	
___	___	___	18. Apply Betadine ointment to insertion site.	

Procedure 27-4

Administering Total Parenteral Nutrition (TPN) (continued)

Excellent ▼	Satisfactory ▼	Needs Practice ▼		COMMENTS
——	——	——	19. Loosen tubing at catheter hub.	
——	——	——	20. Ask patient to hold breath and bear down (Valsalva) while quickly disconnecting old tubing and attaching new tubing to catheter hub.	
——	——	——	21. Tape all connections.	
——	——	——	22. Place transparent, semipermeable dressing over insertion site. (Optional: Paint skin margins with tincture of Benzoin before placing dressing to ensure a tighter seal.)	
——	——	——	23. Loop and tape tubing next to dressing.	
——	——	——	24. Label dressing and tubing with date and your name.	
——	——	——	25. Adjust flow rate per physician's order.	
——	——	——	26. Discard used solution and tubing. Remove gloves.	
——	——	——	27. Document tubing change on client's record and amount infused on intake and output record.	

Administering Intralipids

——	——	——	1. Check solution against physician's order. Inspect solution for separation of emulsion into layers or for froth. Do not use if present.	
——	——	——	2. Wash hands.	
——	——	——	3. Attach fat emulsion tubing to bottle. Prime tubing as for a conventional IV.	
——	——	——	4. Place 19- or 21-gauge one-inch needle on distal end of tubing.	
——	——	——	5. Identify client.	
——	——	——	6. Identify Y-port on hyperalimentation tubing (below in-line filter).	
——	——	——	7. Cleanse Y-port with antiseptic swab. Allow to dry. Insert needle into port. Secure with tape.	
——	——	——	8. Adjust flow rate to infuse at 1.0 mL/minute for adults and 0.1 mL/minute for children. Infuse at this rate for 30 minutes while monitoring client and vital signs every 10 minutes.	
——	——	——	9. If adverse reactions occur, stop infusion and notify physician.	

Procedure 27-4

Administering Total Parenteral Nutrition (TPN) (continued)

Excellent	Satisfactory	Needs Practice		COMMENTS
▼	▼	▼		
___	___	___	10. If no adverse reactions occur, adjust flow rate:	
___	___	___	a. Adults: 500 mL intralipid over 4–6 hours.	
___	___	___	b. Children: up to one g/kg over 4 hours.	
___	___	___	11. Document procedure according to agency policy.	

52

Procedure Checklists to Accompany Craven/Hirnle's Fundamentals of Nursing: Human Health and Function, third edition.

Name _____ Date _____

Unit _____ Position _____

Instructor/Evaluator _____ Position _____

Excellent	Satisfactory	Needs Practice	

Procedure 27-5

Administering a Blood Transfusion

Goal: To replace blood volume or blood components lost through trauma, surgery, or a disease process.

COMMENTS

1. Gather equipment. Wash hands. Explain procedure to client. Have client sign consent form, if required by agency policy.

2. Obtain client's vital signs, including temperature.

3. With another RN at client's bedside, verify the blood product and the client's identity by comparing the laboratory blood record with:

   a. Client's name and identification number, both verbally and against client's wristband.

   b. Blood unit number on the blood bag label.

   c. Blood group and RH type on the blood bag label.

   d. Verify the type of blood component and the expiration date noted on the blood label.

   e. Document verification by both RN signatures on transfusion record.

4. Wash hands.

5. Open Y-type blood administration set and clamp both rollers completely.

6. Spike 0.9% NaCl container. Prime drip chamber and tubing with saline.

7. Spike blood or blood component unit with second spike. Keep roller clamp shut.

8. Remove primary IV tubing from catheter hub and cover end with sterile protector.

9. Attach blood administration tubing to catheter hub and secure with tape.

Copyright © 2000 by Lippincott Williams & Wilkins. Procedure Checklists to Accompany Craven/Hirnle's *Fundamentals of Nursing: Human Health and Function,* third edition by Elissa Swisher Sauer

Procedure 27-5

Administering a Blood Transfusion (continued)

Excellent ▼	Satisfactory ▼	Needs Practice ▼		COMMENTS
___	___	___	10. Flush line with normal saline. Open clamp to blood product. Open roller clamp below drip chamber and begin transfusion.	
___	___	___	11. Infuse blood slowly for first 15 minutes at 10 drops per minute.	
___	___	___	12. Monitor and document vital signs every 5 minutes during first 15 minutes, assessing for chilling, back pain, headache, nausea or vomiting, tachycardia, hypotension, tachypnea, or skin rash.	
___	___	___	13. If adverse reactions occur, close clamp to blood, open clamp to 0.9% NaCl, and notify physician immediately. Follow agency policy for laboratory notification and obtaining blood and urine specimens.	
___	___	___	14. If no adverse reactions occur after 15 minutes, regulate clamp to increase infusion according to physician's order. A unit of blood is usually administered over 2 hours. Monitor vital signs hourly until transfusion is complete.	
___	___	___	15. When blood transfusion is complete, clamp roller to blood and open roller to 0.9% NaCl solution. Infuse until tubing is clear.	
___	___	___	16. Obtain and document posttransfusion vital signs.	
___	___	___	17. If second blood component unit is to be transfused, slow 0.9% NaCl solution to keep vein open until next unit is available. Follow verification procedure and vital sign monitoring for each unit.	
___	___	___	18. If transfusion orders are complete, disconnect the blood administration tubing from catheter hub. Reconnect primary intravenous solution and tubing and adjust to desired rate.	
___	___	___	19. Wash hands.	
___	___	___	20. Document procedure on client's record.	

Procedure Checklists to Accompany Craven/Hirnle's Fundamentals of Nursing: Human Health and Function, third edition.

Name _____ Date _____

Unit _____ Position _____

Instructor/Evaluator _____ Position _____

Excellent ▼	Satisfactory ▼	Needs Practice ▼	
			## Procedure 31-1 # Assisting with the Bath or Shower **Goal:** To cleanse the skin, stimulate circulation, control body odors, and promote self-esteem.
			COMMENTS
——	——	——	1. Make sure tub and shower are clean.
——	——	——	2. Place towel or disposable bath mat on floor by tub or shower.
——	——	——	3. Don gloves.
——	——	——	4. Accompany or transport client to bathroom. Use shower chair, if indicated.
——	——	——	5. Place "Occupied" sign on bathroom door.
——	——	——	6. Keep client covered with bath blanket until water is ready.
——	——	——	7. Fill bathtub halfway with warm water (105°F). Test water or have client test water. If client is showering, turn shower on and adjust temperature.
——	——	——	8. Help client into shower or tub, providing necessary assistance.
——	——	——	9. Instruct client to use safety bars and call-bell signal. Client may prefer to sit in shower chair to prevent fatigue.
——	——	——	10. If client is unable to shower independently, stay with client at all times. Use hand-held shower to wash client.
——	——	——	11. If client is showering or bathing independently, check on client within 15 minutes. Wash any areas he or she could not reach.
——	——	——	12. Help client out of tub or shower. Assist with drying.
——	——	——	13. If client is unsteady, drain water before getting client out of tub to prevent falls.
——	——	——	14. Assist client with dressing and grooming.

Excellent	Satisfactory	Needs Practice	
▼	▼	▼	

Procedure 31-1
Assisting with the Bath or Shower (continued)

COMMENTS

___	___	___	15. Help client to room.
___	___	___	16. Return to bathroom to clean tub or shower according to agency policy. Discard soiled linen. Place "Unoccupied" sign on door.

Procedure Checklists to Accompany Craven/Hirnle's Fundamentals of Nursing: Human Health and Function, third edition.

Name _____ Date _____

Unit _____ Position _____

Instructor/Evaluator _____ Position _____

Excellent ▼	Satisfactory ▼	Needs Practice ▼	
			Procedure 31-2
			Bathing a Client in Bed
			Goal: To cleanse the skin, stimulate circulation, control body odors, and promote self-esteem.

COMMENTS

Excellent	Satisfactory	Needs Practice	
___	___	___	1. Close curtains around bed or shut room door.
___	___	___	2. Help client to use bedpan, urinal, or commode, if needed.
___	___	___	3. Close window and doors to decrease drafts.
___	___	___	4. Wash your hands.
___	___	___	5. Raise bed to high position. Lock side rail up on opposite side of bed from your work.
___	___	___	6. Remove top sheet and bedspread and place bath blanket on client. Help client move closer to you, and remove client's gown. If reusing top linen, place it on back of chair; otherwise, place in laundry bag. If client has an IV line, remove gown from arm, lower IV container, and slide it through gown with tubing. Rehang IV container and check flow rate.
___	___	___	7. Lay towel across patient's chest.
___	___	___	8. Wet washcloth and fold around your finger to make a mitt:
___	___	___	a. Fold washcloth in thirds.
___	___	___	b. Straighten washcloth to take out wrinkles.
___	___	___	c. Fold washcloth over to fit hand.
___	___	___	d. Tuck loose ends under edge of washcloth on palm.
___	___	___	9. Cleanse eyes with water only, wiping from inner to outer canthus. Use separate corner of mitt for each eye.
___	___	___	10. Determine if client would like soap used on face. Wash face, neck, and ears.
___	___	___	11. Fold bath blanket off arm away from you. Place towel lengthwise under arm. Wash, rinse, and dry the arm using long, firm strokes from fingers toward axilla. Wash axilla.

Excellent ▼	Satisfactory ▼	Needs Practice ▼	*Procedure 31-2* **Bathing a Client in Bed (continued)**
			COMMENTS
___	___	___	12. (Optional) Place bath towel on bed and put wash basin on it. Immerse client's hand and allow to soak for several minutes. Wash, rinse, and dry hand well. Repeat on other side. Apply lotion.
___	___	___	13. Repeat for arm and hand nearest you.
___	___	___	14. Apply deodorant or powder according to client's preferences. Avoid excessive use of powder or inhalation of powder.
___	___	___	15. Assess temperature of bath water and change water if necessary. If you leave bedside, lock side rails up to prevent accidental falls.
___	___	___	16. Place bath towel over chest. Fold bath blanket down to below umbilicus.
___	___	___	17. Lift bath towel off chest and bathe chest and abdomen with mitted hand using long, firm strokes. Give special attention to skin under breasts and any other skin folds, if client is overweight. Rinse and dry well.
___	___	___	18. Help client don clean gown.
___	___	___	19. Expose leg away from you by folding over bath blanket. Be careful to keep perineum covered.
___	___	___	20. Lift leg and place bath towel lengthwise under leg. Wash, rinse, and dry leg using long, firm strokes from ankle to thigh.
___	___	___	21. Wash feet or place in basin of water as for hands. Rinse and dry well. Pay special attention to space between toes.
___	___	___	22. Repeat for other leg and foot.
___	___	___	23. Assess bath water for warmth. Change water if necessary.
___	___	___	24. Assist client to side-lying position. Place bath towel along side of back and buttocks to protect linen. Wash, rinse, and dry back and buttocks. Give back rub with powder or lotion.
___	___	___	25. Assist to supine position. Assess if client can wash genitals and perineal area independently. If unable, drape client with bath blanket so that only genitals are exposed. Don disposable, clean gloves; using fresh water and a new cloth, wash, rinse, and dry genitalia and perineum.
___	___	___	26. Apply powder, lotion, or cologne according to client preference.

Excellent	Satisfactory	Needs Practice		
▼	▼	▼		

Procedure 31-2

Bathing a Client in Bed (continued)

COMMENTS

Excellent	Satisfactory	Needs Practice		
____	____	____	27. Assist with hair and mouth care.	
____	____	____	28. Make bed with clean linen.	
____	____	____	29. Clean equipment and return to appropriate storage area.	
____	____	____	30. Wash your hands.	
____	____	____	31. Chart significant observations.	

Procedure Checklists to Accompany Craven/Hirnle's Fundamentals of Nursing: Human Health and Function, third edition.

Name _____ Date _____

Unit _____ Position _____

Instructor/Evaluator _____ Position _____

Excellent	Satisfactory	Needs Practice	*Procedure 31-3* **Massaging the Back**	COMMENTS
			Goal: To stimulate circulation to the skin and promote comfort and relaxation.	
___	___	___	1. Help client to side-lying or prone position.	
___	___	___	2. Expose back, shoulders, upper arms, and sacral area. Cover remainder of body with bath blanket.	
___	___	___	3. Wash hands in warm water. Warm lotion by holding container under running, warm water.	
___	___	___	4. Pour small amount of lotion into palms.	
___	___	___	5. Begin massage in sacral area with circular motion. Move hands upward to shoulders, massaging over scapulae in smooth, firm strokes. Without removing hands from skin, continue in smooth strokes to upper arms and down sides of back to iliac crest. Continue for 3–5 minutes.	
___	___	___	6. While massaging, assess for whitish or reddened areas that do not disappear, and broken skin areas. Avoid pressure over areas of breakdown or redness.	
___	___	___	7. If additional stimulation is desired, petrissage (kneading) over shoulders and gluteal area and tapotement (tapping) up and down spine is done.	
___	___	___	8. End massage with long, continuous stroking movements.	
___	___	___	9. Pat excess lubricant dry with towel. Retie gown and assist client to comfortable position.	
___	___	___	10. Wash hands.	

60

Procedure Checklists to Accompany Craven/Hirnle's Fundamentals of Nursing: Human Health and Function, third edition.

Name _____ Date _____

Unit _____ Position _____

Instructor/Evaluator _____ Position _____

Excellent	Satisfactory	Needs Practice	*Procedure 31-4* **Performing Foot and Nail Care**	COMMENTS
▼	▼	▼	**Goal:** To maintain skin integrity around nails and maintain foot function.	
___	___	___	1. Wash hands.	
___	___	___	2. Help patient to chair, if possible. Elevate head of bed for bedridden client.	
___	___	___	3. Remove colored nail polish if client is scheduled for surgery. Review agency policy to determine if client may wear clear nail polish.	
___	___	___	4. Fill washbasin with warm water (100°–104°F). Place waterproof pad under basin. Soak client's hands or feet in basin.	
___	___	___	5. Place call bell within reach. Allow hands or feet to soak for 10–20 minutes.	
___	___	___	6. Dry hand or foot that has been soaking. Rewarm water and allow other extremity to soak while you work on the softened nails.	
___	___	___	7. Gently clean under nails with orange stick. If nails are thickened and yellow, client may have fungal infection. Don disposable, clean gloves to prevent transmission of infection.	
___	___	___	8. Beginning with large toe or thumb, clip nail straight across. Shape nail with file. File rather than cut nails of clients with diabetes or circulatory problems.	
___	___	___	9. Refer patient with severely hypertrophied nails to podiatrist or foot clinic.	
___	___	___	10. Push cuticle back gently with orange stick.	
___	___	___	11. Repeat procedure with other nails.	
___	___	___	12. Rinse foot or hand in warm water.	
___	___	___	13. Dry thoroughly with towel, especially between digits.	

Copyright © 2000 by Lippincott Williams & Wilkins. Procedure Checklists to Accompany Craven/Hirnle's *Fundamentals of Nursing: Human Health and Function,* third edition by Elissa Swisher Sauer

Excellent ▼	Satisfactory ▼	Needs Practice ▼	*Procedure 31-4* **Performing Foot and Nail Care (continued)**	COMMENTS
____	____	____	14. Apply lotion to hands or feet.	
____	____	____	15. Help client to comfortable position.	
____	____	____	16. Remove and dispose of equipment.	
____	____	____	17. Wash hands.	

62

Name _____ Date _____

Unit _____ Position _____

Instructor/Evaluator _____ Position _____

Excellent	Satisfactory	Needs Practice	*Procedure 31-5* **Shampooing Hair of Bedridden Client**	
▼	▼	▼	**Goal:** To cleanse hair and scalp.	**COMMENTS**
___	___	___	1. Place waterproof pads under client's head and shoulders and remove pillow.	
___	___	___	2. Raise bed to highest position.	
___	___	___	3. Remove any pins from hair. Comb and brush hair thoroughly.	
___	___	___	4. Lay bed to flat position.	
___	___	___	5. Place shampooing basin under head. Place bath towel around shoulders and folded washcloth where neck rests on basin.	
___	___	___	6. Fold bed linens down to waist. Cover upper body with bath blanket.	
___	___	___	7. Place waste basket with plastic bag under spout of shampoo basin on a chair or table at the bedside.	
___	___	___	8. Using water pitcher, wet hair thoroughly with warm water (approximately 110°F). Check temperature by placing small amount of water on your wrist or with bath thermometer.	
___	___	___	9. Apply small amount of shampoo. If needed, use hydrogen peroxide to dissolve matted blood in hair. Reassure client it will not bleach the hair.	
___	___	___	10. Massage scalp with fingertips while making shampoo lather. Start at hairline and work toward neck.	
___	___	___	11. Rinse hair with warm water. Reapply shampoo and repeat massage.	
___	___	___	12. Rinse hair thoroughly with warm water.	
___	___	___	13. Apply small amount of conditioner per patient request. Rinse well.	

Procedure 31-5
Shampooing Hair of Bedridden Client (continued)

Excellent	Satisfactory	Needs Practice		COMMENTS
▼	▼	▼		
___	___	___	14. Squeeze excess moisture from hair. Wrap bath towel around hair. Rub to dry hair and scalp. Use second towel if necessary.	
___	___	___	15. Remove equipment and wet towels from bed. Place dry towel around client's shoulders.	
___	___	___	16. Dry hair with hair dryer. Comb and style.	
___	___	___	17. Help client to comfortable position.	
___	___	___	18. Dispose of soiled equipment and linen.	

Procedure Checklists to Accompany Craven/Hirnle's Fundamentals of Nursing: Human Health and Function, third edition.

Name _____ Date _____

Unit _____ Position _____

Instructor/Evaluator _____ Position _____

Excellent	Satisfactory	Needs Practice	
▼	▼	▼	***Procedure 31-6*** **Providing Oral Care** **Goal:** To cleanse tooth and mouth surfaces to prevent odor and caries.

COMMENTS

____	____	____	1. Wash hands.
____	____	____	2. Close bedside curtains or room door and explain procedure to client.
____	____	____	3. Help client to a sitting position. If client cannot sit, help to a side-lying position.
____	____	____	4. Place towel under client's chin.
____	____	____	5. Moisten toothbrush with water. Apply small amount of toothpaste.
____	____	____	6. Hand toothbrush to client or don disposable gloves and brush client's teeth as follows:
____	____	____	a. Hold toothbrush at a 45-degree angle to gum line.
____	____	____	b. Using short, vibrating motions, brush from gum line to crown of each tooth. Repeat until outside and inside of teeth and gums are cleaned.
____	____	____	c. Cleanse biting surfaces by brushing with back-and-forth stroke.
____	____	____	d. Brush tongue lightly. Avoid stimulating the gag reflex.
____	____	____	7. Have client rinse mouth thoroughly with water and spit into emesis basin.
____	____	____	8. Remove emesis basin, set aside, and dry client's mouth with washcloth.
____	____	____	9. Floss client's teeth:
____	____	____	a. Cut 10-inch piece of dental floss. Wind ends of floss around middle finger of each hand.
____	____	____	b. Using index fingers to stretch the floss, move the floss up and down around and between lower teeth. Start at the back lower teeth and work around to other side.

Excellent	Satisfactory	Needs Practice	
▼	▼	▼	*Procedure 31-6* **Providing Oral Care (continued)** COMMENTS
___	___	___	c. Using thumb and index fingers to stretch floss, repeat procedure on upper teeth.
___	___	___	d. Have client rinse mouth thoroughly and spit into emesis basin.
___	___	___	10. Remove basin. Dry client's mouth.
___	___	___	11. Remove and dispose of supplies. Help client to comfortable position.
___	___	___	12. Wash hands.
			Variations for the Unconscious Client
___	___	___	1. Gather equipment.
___	___	___	2. Place client in a side-lying position with head of bed lowered so saliva runs out of mouth by gravity.
___	___	___	3. Place towel or waterproof pad under client's chin.
___	___	___	4. Place emesis basin against client's mouth, or have suction catheter positioned to remove secretions from mouth.
___	___	___	5. Use padded tongue blade to open teeth gently. Leave in place between the back molars. Never put your fingers in an unconscious client's mouth.
___	___	___	6. Brush teeth and gums as directed preciously, using toothbrush or soft sponge-ended swab.
___	___	___	7. Swab or suction to remove pooled secretions. A small bulb syringe or syringe without a needle may be used to rinse oral cavity.
___	___	___	8. Apply thin layer of petroleum jelly to lips to prevent drying or cracking. Note: Lemon and glycerine swabs can cause drying to oral mucosa if used for extended periods.

Procedure Checklists to Accompany Craven/Hirnle's Fundamentals of Nursing: Human Health and Function, third edition.

Name _____ Date _____

Unit _____ Position _____

Instructor/Evaluator _____ Position _____

Excellent ▼	Satisfactory ▼	Needs Practice ▼	

Procedure 31-7

Using a Bedpan

Goal: To provide a means of elimination for clients who are confined to bed or are unable to get to the bathroom or bedside commode.

COMMENTS

Placing the Bedpan

1. Wash hands. Don clean gloves.

2. Close curtain around bed or shut door.

3. Run warm water over rim of pan; dry with towel.

4. Position and lock side rail up on opposite side of bed from which you work.

5. Raise bed to height appropriate for nurse.

6. If client can raise buttocks and assist:

   a. Fold top linen down on nurse's side to expose patient's hips.

   b. Have client flex knees and lift buttocks. Assist by placing your hand under sacrum, elbow on mattress, and lifting as a lever.

   c. Slide rounded, smooth rim of regular bedpan under client. If using fracture pan, slide narrow, flat end under buttocks.

7. If client is unable to assist by raising buttocks:

   a. Lower head of bed to flat position.

   b. Fold top linens down to expose client minimally.

   c. Help client to roll to side-lying position.

   d. Place bedpan against buttocks and tucked down against mattress. Hold firmly in place and roll patient onto back as bedpan is positioned under buttocks.

8. Cover client with linen. Place call bell and toilet paper within reach.

Procedure 31-7

Using a Bedpan (continued)

Excellent	Satisfactory	Needs Practice		COMMENTS
▼	▼	▼		
___	___	___	9. Raise head of bed 45–80 degress unless contraindicated.	
___	___	___	10. Lower bed to lowest position. Place side rails up if indicated.	
___	___	___	11. Wash hands. Allow client to be alone.	
			Removing the Bedpan	
___	___	___	12. Answer call bell promptly.	
___	___	___	13. Place soap, wet washcloth, and towel at bedside.	
___	___	___	14. Raise bed to appropriate working height for nurse.	
___	___	___	15. Fold back top linens to expose patient minimally.	
___	___	___	16. Put on disposable clean gloves.	
___	___	___	17. Assess if client can wipe perineal area. If not, wipe area with several layers of toilet tissue. If specimen is to be measured or collected, dispose of soiled toilet tissue in separate receptacle, not in bedpan. (For female clients, wipe from urethra to anus.)	
___	___	___	18. If client can raise buttocks and assist with procedure:	
___	___	___	a. Lower head of bed.	
___	___	___	b. Have client flex knees and lift buttocks. Assist by placing one hand under sacrum and supporting bedpan with other hand to prevent spillage. Remove bedpan and place on bedside chair.	
___			c. Offer soap, warm water, washcloth, and towel for client to wash hands and/or perineal area.	
___	___	___	19. If client is unable to assist by raising buttocks:	
___	___	___	a. Lower head of bed to flat position.	
___	___	___	b. Fold top linen down to expose patient minimally.	
___	___	___	c. Help client to roll off bedpan and onto side. Use one hand to stabilize bedpan during turning to prevent spillage.	
___	___	___	d. Wipe anal area with tissue. Wash perineum with soap and warm water. Pat dry.	
___	___	___	20. Assist client to comfortable position.	

Procedure 31-7
Using a Bedpan (continued)

Excellent	Satisfactory	Needs Practice		COMMENTS
—	—	—	21. Cover bedpan and remove from bedside. Obtain specimen if required. Empty and clean bedpan and return it to bedside.	
—	—	—	22. Remove and discard gloves. Wash hands.	
—	—	—	23. Spray air freshener if necessary to control odor, unless contraindicated (respiratory conditions, allergies).	

Procedure Checklists to Accompany Craven/Hirnle's Fundamentals of Nursing: Human Health and Function, third edition.

Name _____ Date _____

Unit _____ Position _____

Instructor/Evaluator _____ Position _____

Excellent	Satisfactory	Needs Practice	*Procedure 31-8* **Making an Unoccupied Bed**	COMMENTS
▼	▼	▼	**Goal:** To provide clean linen and remove sources of skin irritation.	
___	___	___	1. Wash hands.	
___	___	___	2. Assemble equipment on bedside table or chair.	
___	___	___	3. Help client to chair at bedside.	
___	___	___	4. Raise bed to comfortable working position.	
___	___	___	5. Loosen linen on one side of bed. Move to other side of bed and loosen all linen.	
___	___	___	6. Remove bedspread and blanket and fold each separately if they are to be reused. Place over back of chair.	
___	___	___	7. Remove pillowcases by grasping seamed end with one hand and pulling pillow out with the other. Place pillows on chair. Discard pillowcases in linen bag.	
___	___	___	8. Remove each piece of linen separately by rolling into a ball and discarding into linen bag. Be careful to prevent soiled linen from touching your uniform.	
___	___	___	9. Slide mattress to head of bed if it has slipped to the foot.	
___	___	___	10. Wipe mattress with antiseptic solution if grossly soiled. Dry thoroughly.	
___	___	___	11. Working from side of bed where linen is stored, spread mattress pad over mattress and smooth out wrinkles.	
___	___	___	12. Unfold bottom sheet lengthwise on bed with vertical center crease along center of bed. Unfold top layer toward opposite side of mattress. Pull remaining top sheet over head of mattress, leaving bottom edge of sheet even with mattress edge. Smooth bottom sheet with hand.	
___	___	___	13. Standing near head of bed, tuck excess sheet under the mattress on your side at the end of the bed.	

Excellent	Satisfactory	Needs Practice	

Procedure 31-8
Making an Unoccupied Bed (continued)

COMMENTS

Excellent	Satisfactory	Needs Practice	
—	—	—	14. Miter the corner on your side:
—	—	—	a. Grasp side edge of sheet about 18 inches down from mattress top.
—	—	—	b. Lay sheet on top of mattress to form triangular, flat fold.
—	—	—	c. Tuck sheet hanging loose below mattress under the mattress, without pulling on triangular fold.
—	—	—	d. Pick up top of triangular fold and place it over side of mattress.
			e. Tuck this loose portion of sheet under mattress.
—	—	—	15. Tuck remaining sheet on that side under the mattress.
—	—	—	16. Lay draw sheet, folded in half, on the bed with the center fold at center of bed. Place top edge of draw sheet about 12–15 inches from head of bed. Tuck excess draw sheet under mattress.
—	—	—	17. Move to opposite side of bed.
—	—	—	18. Spread bottom sheet over mattress edge and miter top corner.
—	—	—	19. Tuck excess bottom sheet tightly under mattress, pulling gently to smooth out wrinkles.
—	—	—	20. Grasp draw sheet, pulling gently. Beginning at middle, tuck draw sheet under mattress firmly. Finish tucking top and bottom.
—	—	—	21. Return to side of bed where linen is placed.
—	—	—	22. Place top sheet on bed with vertical center fold at center of bed. Unfold sheet with seams facing out and top edge even with top of mattress. Smooth sheet, with excess falling over bottom edge of mattress.
—	—	—	23. Spread blanket and bedspread evenly over bed.
—	—	—	24. Miter the bottom corner, using all three layers of linen (sheet, blanket, bedspread). Leave sides untucked.
—	—	—	25. Move to opposite side of bed and miter bottom corner, using all three linen layers.
—	—	—	26. Standing at bottom of bed, grasp top covers about 10 inches from bottom of mattress. Loosen linen slightly by pulling on top covers or forming a pleat.

Procedure 31-8

Making an Unoccupied Bed (continued)

Excellent	Satisfactory	Needs Practice	
▼	▼	▼	COMMENTS

___	___	___	27. Put on clean pillowcases:
___	___	___	a. Grasp center of pillowcase, with one hand on seamed end.
___	___	___	b. Gather case, turning it inside out over the hand holding it.
___	___	___	c. With same hand, grasp middle of one end of pillow.
___	___	___	d. Pull case over pillow with free hand.
___	___	___	e. Adjust case so corners fit over pillow.
___	___	___	28. Place pillows in center at head of bed.
___	___	___	29. Fold top linen back to one side or fanfold at bottom of bed.
___	___	___	30. Secure call bell within patient's reach and lower bed.
___	___	___	31. Arrange bedside table, nightstand, and personal items within easy reach.
___	___	___	32. Discard soiled linen according to agency policy.
___	___	___	33. Wash hands.

Procedure Checklists to Accompany Craven/Hirnle's Fundamentals of Nursing: Human Health and Function, third edition.

Name _____ Date _____

Unit _____ Position _____

Instructor/Evaluator _____ Position _____

Excellent	Satisfactory	Needs Practice	

Procedure 31-9
Making an Occupied Bed

Goal: To provide clean linen for client who is unable to get out of bed.

COMMENTS

1. Wash hands.
2. Assemble equipment on bedside table or chair.
3. Close door or bedside curtains.
4. Lock side rails up on side of bed opposite from where clean linen is stacked.
5. Raise bed to comfortable working position. Lower side rail on your side of bed.
6. Loosen all top linen from foot of bed.
7. Remove bedspread and blanket separately. Without shaking, fold each and place over back of chair if they are to be reused. If they are soiled, hold them away from your uniform and place in linen bag.
8. Leave top sheet on client or cover client with a bath blanket, then remove and discard top sheet.
9. Loosen bottom sheet on your side.
10. Lower head of bed to flat position. If client cannot tolerate flat position, lower head of bed as far as client can tolerate.
11. With assistance from another worker, grasp mattress lugs and slide mattress to head of bed if it has slipped down.
12. Help client roll onto side facing away from you. Have client grasp side rail to assist. Adjust pillow under head.
13. Tightly fan-fold soiled draw sheet and tuck under buttocks, back, and shoulders. Repeat with soiled bottom sheet and tuck under client. Do not fan-fold mattress pad unless it is soiled.

Excellent	Satisfactory	Needs Practice		COMMENTS
			Procedure 31-9 **Making an Occupied Bed (continued)**	
___	___	___	14. Place clean bottom sheet on bed. Unfold lengthwise so bottom edge is even with end of mattress and vertical center crease is at center of bed.	
___	___	___	15. Bring sheet's bottom edge over mattress sides and fanfold top of sheet toward center of mattress and place tightly next to patient.	
___	___	___	16. Tuck top edge of sheet under mattress. Miter the corner on your side (as in Procedure 31-8) and tuck remaining portion of sheet under mattress. Note: If contour sheets are used, fit elastic edges under corner of mattress.	
___	___	___	17. Place draw sheet on bed with the center fold at center of bed. Position sheet so it will extend from patient's back to below the buttocks. Fan-fold the top edge and place next to client. Tuck excess under mattress.	
___	___	___	18. Lock side rails up and move to opposite side of bed.	
___	___	___	19. Lower side rail. Help client roll over folds of linen onto other side.	
___	___	___	20. Move pillow under client's head.	
___	___	___	21. Remove soiled linen by folding into a square or bundle, with soiled side turned in. Place in linen bag.	
___	___	___	22. Grasp edge of fan-folded bottom sheet and pull from under client.	
___	___	___	23. Tuck top of sheet under top of mattress. Miter top corner.	
___	___	___	24. Facing bed, pull bottom sheet tight and tuck excess linen under mattress from top to bottom.	
___	___	___	25. Unfold draw sheet by grasping at center. Tuck excess tightly under mattress. Tuck the middle first, then the top, and finally the bottom.	
___	___	___	26. Help client to center of bed.	
___	___	___	27. Raise side rail if necessary and move to side of bed where remainder of linen is stored.	
___	___	___	28. Place top sheet over client with center crease lengthwise at center of bed with seam side up. Unfold sheet from head to toe.	
___	___	___	29. Have client grasp top edge of clean top sheet. Remove bath blanket or soiled top linen by pulling from beneath clean top sheet.	

Procedure 31-9

Making an Occupied Bed (continued)

Excellent ▼	Satisfactory ▼	Needs Practice ▼		COMMENTS
——	——	——	30. Discard in linen bag.	
——	——	——	31. Complete top covers as described in Procedure 31-8.	
——	——	——	32. Wash hands.	

75

Procedure Checklists to Accompany Craven/Hirnle's Fundamentals of Nursing: Human Health and Function, third edition.

Name _____ Date _____

Unit _____ Position _____

Instructor/Evaluator _____ Position _____

Excellent	Satisfactory	Needs Practice	Procedure 32-1 — Using Proper Body Mechanics to Move Clients	COMMENTS
▼	▼	▼	**Goal:** To prevent injury to the nurse's musculoskeletal system and to prevent injury to clients during transfer.	
___	___	___	1. Wash hands.	
___	___	___	2. Plan movement before doing it:	
___	___	___	a. Lock wheels on bed, stretcher, or wheelchair.	
___	___	___	b. Allow patient to assist during move.	
___	___	___	c. Use mechanical aids or additional personnel to move heavy clients.	
___	___	___	d. Slide, push, or pull client rather than lifting and carrying, when possible.	
___	___	___	e. Tighten abdominal and gluteal muscles before lifting or moving client.	
___	___	___	f. Use smooth, rhythmic, coordinated movements.	
___	___	___	g. Plan movements before beginning when another person is assisting.	
___	___	___	3. Begin all movements with body aligned and balanced:	
___	___	___	a. Face client to be moved and pivot your entire body without twisting your back.	
___	___	___	b. Place both feet flat on floor, knees slightly bent, with one foot slightly in front of the other or one step apart.	
___	___	___	c. Bend knees to lower center of gravity toward client to be moved.	
___	___	___	4. Elevate adjustable beds to waist level, and lower side rails to prevent stretching.	
___	___	___	5. Carry objects close to body and stand as close as possible to work area.	

Copyright © 2000 by Lippincott Williams & Wilkins. Procedure Checklists to Accompany Craven/Hirnle's *Fundamentals of Nursing: Human Health and Function,* third edition by Elissa Swisher Sauer

Procedure Checklists to Accompany Craven/Hirnle's Fundamentals of Nursing: Human Health and Function, third edition.

Name _____ Date _____

Unit _____ Position _____

Instructor/Evaluator _____ Position _____

Excellent ▼	Satisfactory ▼	Needs Practice ▼	*Procedure 32-2* **Positioning a Client in Bed** **Goal:** To maintain proper body alignment for optimal ventilation and lung expansion, and to prevent deformities of musculo-skeletal system.	COMMENTS
			Moving a Client Up in Bed (One Nurse)	
___	___	___	1. Wash hands. Explain procedure and rationale to client.	
___	___	___	2. Lower head of bed to flat position and raise level of bed to comfortable working height.	
___	___	___	3. Remove all pillows from under client. Leave one at head of bed.	
___	___	___	4. Instruct client to bend legs and put feet flat on bed.	
___	___	___	5. Place your feet in broad stance with one foot in front of the other. Flex your knees and thighs.	
___	___	___	6. Place one arm under client's shoulders and one arm under thighs.	
___	___	___	7. Rock back and forth on front and back legs to count of three. On third count, have client push with feet as you lift and pull client up in bed.	
___	___	___	8. Elevate head of bed and place pillows under head. Raise side rails and lower bed to lowest level.	
			Moving Helpless Client Up in Bed (Two Nurses)	
___	___	___	1. Explain procedure and rationale to client.	
___	___	___	2. Lower head of bed to flat position and raise level of bed to comfortable working height.	
___	___	___	3. Remove all pillows from under client. Leave one at head of bed.	
___	___	___	4. One nurse stands on each side of bed with wide base of support and one foot slightly in front of the other.	
___	___	___	5. Each nurse rolls up and grasps edges of turn sheet close to client's shoulders and buttocks.	

Excellent	Satisfactory	Needs Practice	
▼	▼	▼	

Procedure 32-2

Positioning a Client in Bed (continued)

COMMENTS

——	——	——	6. Flex knees and hips. Tighten abdominal and gluteal muscles and keep back straight.
——	——	——	7. Rock back and forth on front and back leg to count of three. On third count, both nurses shift weight to front leg as they simultaneously lift client toward head of bed.
——	——	——	8. Elevate head of bed and place pillows under client's head. Adjust other positioning pillows as necessary. Put up side rails and lower bed to lowest level.

Positioning Client in Side-Lying Position

——	——	——	1. Lower head of bed as flat as client can tolerate.
——	——	——	2. Elevate and lock side rail on side client will face when turned.
——	——	——	3. Place arm that client will turn toward away from his or her body. Fold other arm across chest.
——	——	——	4. Flex client's knee that will not be next to mattress after turn. Have client reach toward side rail with opposite arm.
——	——	——	5. Assume a broad stance with knees slightly flexed.
——	——	——	6. Using a draw sheet, gently pull client over on side.
——	——	——	7. Align client properly, and place pillows behind back and under head.
——	——	——	8. Pull shoulder blade forward and out from under client. Support client's upper arm with pillow.
——	——	——	9. Place pillow lengthwise between client's legs from thighs to foot.

Logrolling

——	——	——	1. Obtain assistance of two or three other nurses.
——	——	——	2. All nurses stand on same side of bed, with feet apart, one foot slightly ahead of the other. Flex knees and hips.
——	——	——	3. Use one pillow to support client's head during and after turn.
——	——	——	4. Place pillows between client's legs.
——	——	——	5. Instruct client to fold arms over chest and keep body stiff.
——	——	——	6. Reach across client and support head, thorax, trunk, and legs.
——	——	——	7. On count of three, roll client in one coordinated movement to lateral position.

Excellent ▼	Satisfactory ▼	Needs Practice ▼	*Procedure 32-2* **Positioning a Client in Bed (continued)**	
				COMMENTS
___	___	___	8. Support client in alignment with pillows as described in section on "side-lying position." Clients with suspected or known cervical spinal injuries should wear cervical collars to prevent injury to the spinal cord whenever turning or moving in bed.	

Procedure Checklists to Accompany Craven/Hirnle's Fundamentals of Nursing: Human Health and Function, third edition.

Name _____ Date _____

Unit _____ Position _____

Instructor/Evaluator _____ Position _____

Procedure 32-3

Providing Range-of-Motion (ROM) Exercises

Excellent	Satisfactory	Needs Practice		COMMENTS
▼	▼	▼	**Goal:** To maintain joint mobility, improve or maintain muscle strength, and prevent muscle atrophy and contractures.	
___	___	___	1. Wash hands. Explain procedure and purpose to client.	
___	___	___	2. Position client on back with head of bed as flat as possible. Elevate bed to comfortable working height.	
___	___	___	3. Stand on side of bed of joints to be exercised. Uncover only the limb to be exercised.	
___	___	___	4. Perform exercises slowly and gently, providing support by holding areas proximal and distal to the joint.	
___	___	___	5. Repeat each exercise five times. Discontinue or decrease ROM if client complains of discomfort or muscle spasm.	
___	___	___	6. Neck:	
___	___	___	a. Move chin to chest.	
___	___	___	b. Bend head toward back.	
___	___	___	c. Tilt head toward each shoulder.	
___	___	___	d. Rotate head in circular motion.	
___	___	___	e. Return head to erect position.	
___	___	___	7. Shoulder:	
___	___	___	a. Raise client's arm from side to above head.	
___	___	___	b. Abduct and rotate shoulder by raising arm above head with palm up.	
___	___	___	c. Adduct shoulder by moving arm across body as far as possible.	
___	___	___	d. Rotate shoulder internally and externally by flexing elbow and moving forearm so that palm touches mattress; then reverse the motion so that back of client's hand touches mattress.	
___	___	___	e. Move shoulder in a full circle.	

Excellent	Satisfactory	Needs Practice	

Procedure 32-3

Providing Range-of-Motion (ROM) Exercises (continued)

COMMENTS

▼ ▼ ▼

8. Elbow:

   a. Bend elbow so that forearm moves toward shoulder.

   b. Hyperextend elbow as far as possible.

9. Wrist and hand:

   a. Move hand toward inner aspect of forearm.

   b. Bend dorsal surface of hand backward.

   c. Abduct wrist by bending toward thumb.

   d. Adduct wrist by bending toward fifth finger.

   e. Make a fist, then extend the fingers.

   f. Spread fingers apart, then together.

   g. Move thumb across hand to base of fifth finger.

10. Hip and knee:

   a. Lift leg and bend knee toward chest.

   b. Abduct and adduct leg, moving leg laterally away from body and returning to medial position.

   c. Rotate hip internally and externally by turning leg inward, then outward.

   d. Take special care to support joints of larger limbs.

11. Ankle and foot:

   a. Dorsiflex foot by moving foot so toes point upward.

   b. Plantarflex by moving foot so toes point downward.

   c. Curl toes down, then extend.

   d. Spread toes apart, then bring together.

   e. Invert by turning sole of foot medially.

   f. Evert by turning sole of foot laterally.

12. Move to other side of bed and repeat exercises.

13. Reposition client to position of comfort.

14. Wash hands.

15. Document ROM.

Procedure Checklists to Accompany Craven/Hirnle's Fundamentals of Nursing: Human Health and Function, third edition.

Name _____ Date _____

Unit _____ Position _____

Instructor/Evaluator _____ Position _____

Excellent	Satisfactory	Needs Practice	

Procedure 32-4
Assisting with Ambulation

Goal: To promote safe ambulation free of falls or injury.

COMMENTS

1. Wash hands. Explain procedure and purpose of ambulation to client. Decide together how far and where to walk.
2. Place bed in lowest position.
3. Assist client to sitting position on side of bed. Assess for dizziness or faintness. Obtain orthostatic vital signs if patient complains. Allow client to remain in this position until he or she feels secure.
4. Help client with clothing and footwear.

One Nurse

1. Wrap transfer belt around client's waist (optional according to assessment).
2. Assist client to standing position and assess client's balance. Return to bed or transfer to chair if very weak or unsteady. Be sure client does not grasp your neck for support, but places his or her hands around your shoulder or at your waist.
3. Position yourself behind client while supporting him or her by waist or transfer belt.
4. Take several steps forward with client, assessing strength and balance.
5. Encourage client to use good posture and to look ahead, not down at feet.
6. Ambulate for planned distance or time.
7. If client becomes weak or dizzy, return to bed or assist to chair.

Excellent ▼	Satisfactory ▼	Needs Practice ▼	*Procedure 32-4* **Assisting with Ambulation (continued)**
			COMMENTS
___	___	___	8. If client begins to fall, place your feet wide apart with one foot in front. Support client by pulling his or her weight backward against your body. Lower gently to floor, protecting head.
			Two Nurses
___	___	___	1. Assist client to sitting position.
___	___	___	2. Assist client to standing position with one nurse on each side.
___	___	___	3. One nurse grasps the transfer belt to support the client. The other nurse may carry and manage equipment.
___	___	___	4. Walk with client using slow, even steps. Assess strength and balance.
			Using a Walker
___	___	___	1. Assist client to standing position. One hand remains on the arm of the chair or bed as client assumes an upright posture.
___	___	___	2. Have client grasp walker handles.
___	___	___	3. Client moves walker ahead 6–8 inches placing all four feet of walker on floor.
___	___	___	4. Client moves forward to walker.
___	___	___	5. Nurse should walk close behind and slightly to side of client.
___	___	___	6. Repeat above sequence until walk is complete.

Procedure Checklists to Accompany Craven/Hirnle's Fundamentals of Nursing: Human Health and Function, third edition.

Name _____ Date _____

Unit _____ Position _____

Instructor/Evaluator _____ Position _____

Excellent	Satisfactory	Needs Practice	*Procedure 32-5* **Helping Clients with Crutch Walking**	COMMENTS
			Goal: To increase client's level of activity safely after musculoskeletal injury.	
			Four-Point Gait	
___	___	___	1. Wash hands.	
___	___	___	2. Instruct client to stand erect, facing forward in tripod position, placing crutch tips 6 inches in front of feet and 6 inches to side of each foot.	
___	___	___	3. Client moves right crutch forward 6 inches.	
___	___	___	4. Client moves left foot forward to level of right crutch.	
___	___	___	5. Client moves left crutch forward 4–6 inches.	
___	___	___	6. Client moves right foot forward to level of left crutch.	
___	___	___	7. Repeat sequence.	
			Three-Point Gait	
___	___	___	1. Beginning in tripod position, client moves both crutches and affected leg forward.	
___	___	___	2. Client moves stronger leg forward bearing entire weight on stronger leg.	
___	___	___	3. Repeat sequence.	
			Two-Point Gait	
___	___	___	1. Beginning in the tripod position, client moves left crutch and right foot forward.	
___	___	___	2. Client moves right crutch and left foot forward.	
___	___	___	3. Repeat sequence.	

Procedure 32-5

Helping Clients with Crutch Walking (continued)

Excellent ▼	Satisfactory ▼	Needs Practice ▼		COMMENTS
			Swing-to Gait	
___	___	___	1. Client forms tripod position and moves both crutches forward.	
___	___	___	2. Client lifts legs and swings to crutches, supporting body weight on crutches.	
			Climbing Stairs	
___	___	___	1. Use one crutch and the railing. Beginning in tripod position facing stairs, client transfers body weight to crutches and holds onto the railing.	
___	___	___	2. Client places unaffected leg on stair.	
___	___	___	3. Client transfers body weight to unaffected leg.	
___	___	___	4. Client moves crutches and affected leg to stair.	
___	___	___	5. Repeat sequence to top of stairs.	

Procedure Checklists to Accompany Craven/Hirnle's Fundamentals of Nursing: Human Health and Function, third edition.

Name _____ Date _____

Unit _____ Position _____

Instructor/Evaluator _____ Position _____

Excellent	Satisfactory	Needs Practice	*Procedure 32-6* **Transferring a Client to a Stretcher**	COMMENTS
▼	▼	▼	**Goal:** To transfer client without injury to client or nurse.	
___	___	___	1. Wash hands. Explain procedure and purpose to client.	
___	___	___	2. Place stretcher parallel to bed.	
___	___	___	3. Raise bed to same level as stretcher. Lower side rails. Lock wheels on bed.	
___	___	___	4. One or two nurses stand on side of bed without stretcher. Two nurses stand on side of bed with stretcher.	
___	___	___	5. Loosen draw sheet on both sides of bed.	
___	___	___	6. Nurses on side without stretcher help client to move toward them onto his or her side, using draw sheet to pull client closer to stretcher.	
___	___	___	7. Nurses on stretcher side of bed slide transfer board under draw sheet and under client's buttocks and back.	
___	___	___	8. Slide client onto transfer board into supine position. Place client's arms across chest.	
___	___	___	9. Wrap end of draw sheet over curved end of transfer board and slide client onto stretcher on count of three.	
___	___	___	10. Roll client slightly up onto side, and pull transfer board out from under him or her.	
___	___	___	11. Lock side rails up on bed side of stretcher and move stretcher away from bed.	
___	___	___	12. Place sheet over client, and lock safety belts across client's chest and waist. Adjust head of stretcher according to client limitations.	

Procedure Checklists to Accompany Craven/Hirnle's Fundamentals of Nursing: Human Health and Function, third edition.

Name _____   Date _____

Unit _____   Position _____

Instructor/Evaluator _____   Position _____

Procedure 32-7

Transferring a Client to a Wheelchair

Goal: To increase mobility and independence by using wheelchair.

Excellent	Satisfactory	Needs Practice		COMMENTS
▼	▼	▼		
___	___	___	1. Explain procedure to client.	
___	___	___	2. Position wheelchair at 45-degree angle or parallel to bed. Remove footrests and lock brakes.	
___	___	___	3. Lock bed brakes; lower bed to lowest level, and raise head of bed as far as client can tolerate.	
___	___	___	4. Assist client to side-lying position, facing the side of bed on which he or she will sit.	
___	___	___	5. Lower side rail and stand near client's hips with foot near head of bed in front of and apart from other foot.	
___	___	___	6. Apply transfer belt. Grip belt to assist with transfer.	
___	___	___	7. Swing client's legs over side of bed. At the same time, pivot on your back leg to lift client's trunk and shoulders. Keep back straight; avoid twisting.	
___	___	___	8. Stand in front of client and assess for balance and dizziness.	
___	___	___	9. Help client to don robe and nonskid footwear.	
___	___	___	10. Spread your feet apart and flex your hips and knees.	
___	___	___	11. Have client slide buttocks to edge of bed until feet touch floor.	
___	___	___	12. Rock back and forth until client stands on a count of three.	
___	___	___	13. Brace your front knee against client's weak knee as client stands.	
___	___	___	14. Pivot on back foot until client feels wheelchair against back of legs, keeping your knee against the client's knee.	
___	___	___	15. Instruct client to place hands on chair armrests for support. Flex your knees and hips as you assist client into chair.	

Procedure 32-7

Transferring a Client to a Wheelchair (continued)

Excellent	Satisfactory	Needs Practice		COMMENTS
▼	▼	▼		
—	—	—	16. Adjust foot pedal and leg supports.	
—	—	—	17. Assess client's alignment in chair, and secure with restraints as necessary.	

Procedure Checklists to Accompany Craven/Hirnle's Fundamentals of Nursing: Human Health and Function, third edition.

Name _____   Date _____

Unit _____   Position _____

Instructor/Evaluator _____   Position _____

Excellent	Satisfactory	Needs Practice	
▼	▼	▼	**Procedure 33-1** **Monitoring with Pulse Oximetry** **Goal:** To monitor arterial oxygen saturation (SaO_2) noninvasively and to detect deviations from normal promptly.

COMMENTS

____	____	____	1. Select appropriate type of sensor, considering client's weight, level of activity, whether infection control is a concern, allergies, and the anticipated duration of monitoring.
____	____	____	2. Explain purpose of procedure to client and family.
____	____	____	3. Instruct client to breathe normally.
____	____	____	4. Select appropriate site to place sensor. Avoid using lower extremities that have compromised circulation or extremities receiving infusions or other invasive monitoring. Consider use of nasal sensor for clients with poor tissue perfusion.
____	____	____	5. Remove nail polish or acrylic nail from digit to be used.
____	____	____	6. Attach sensor probe and connect it to pulse oximeter. Make sure the photosensors are accurately aligned.
____	____	____	7. Watch for pulse sensing bar on face of oximeter to fluctuate with each pulsation and reflect pulse strength. Double-check machine pulsations with client's radial or apical pulse.
____	____	____	8. If continuous pulse oximetry is desired, set the alarm limits on the monitor to reflect the high and low oxygen saturation *and* pulse rates. Ensure that the alarms are audible before leaving client. Inspect sensor site every 4 hours for tissue irritation or pressure.
____	____	____	9. Read saturation on monitor and document as appropriate with all relevant information on client's chart.
____	____	____	10. Report SaO_2 less than 93% to physician.

Procedure Checklists to Accompany Craven/Hirnle's Fundamentals of Nursing: Human Health and Function, third edition.

Name _____ Date _____

Unit _____ Position _____

Instructor/Evaluator _____ Position _____

Excellent ▼	Satisfactory ▼	Needs Practice ▼	*Procedure 33-2* **Teaching Coughing and Deep-Breathing Exercises** **Goal:** To facilitate respiratory functioning by increasing lung expansion, preventing alveolar collapse, and promoting expectoration of secretions.	COMMENTS
			Deep Breathing	
___	___	___	1. Assist client to Fowler's or sitting position.	
___	___	___	2. Have client place hands palm down, with middle fingers touching, along lower border of rib cage.	
___	___	___	3. Ask client to inhale slowly through the nose, feeling middle fingers separate. Hold breath for 2 or 3 seconds.	
___	___	___	4. Have client exhale slowly through mouth. Repeat three–five times.	
			Controlled Coughing	
___	___	___	1. If adventitious breath sounds or sputum are present, have client take a deep breath, hold for 3 seconds and cough deeply two or three times. Stand to the client's side to ensure the cough is not directed at you. Client must cough deeply, not just clear throat.	
___	___	___	2. If client has an abdominal or chest incision that will be painful during coughing, instruct client to hold a pillow firmly over the incision (splinting) when coughing.	
___	___	___	3. Instruct, reinforce, and supervise deep-breathing and coughing exercises every 2–3 hours postoperatively.	
___	___	___	4. Document procedure.	

Procedure Checklists to Accompany Craven/Hirnle's Fundamentals of Nursing: Human Health and Function, third edition.

Name ______________________________ Date ______________

Unit ______________________________ Position ______________

Instructor/Evaluator ______________________________ Position ______________

Procedure 33-3

Promoting Breathing with the Incentive Spirometer

Goal: To improve pulmonary ventilation and oxygenation and to loosen respiratory secretions.

Excellent	Satisfactory	Needs Practice	Step	COMMENTS
___	___	___	1. Wash hands.	
___	___	___	2. Assist client to high Fowler's on sitting position.	
___	___	___	3. Determine the volume to set incentive spirometry goal based on calculated lung volumes. Use chart or have Respiratory Therapy calculate. Set volume indicator.	
___	___	___	4. Instruct client in procedure:	
___	___	___	a. Seal lips tightly around mouthpiece.	
___	___	___	b. Inhale slowly and deeply through mouth. Hold breath for 2 or 3 seconds.	
___	___	___	c. Have client observe his or her progress by watching the balls elevate or lights go on, depending on type of equipment used.	
___	___	___	d. Exhale slowly around mouthpiece.	
___	___	___	e. Breathe normally for several breaths.	
___	___	___	5. Repeat procedure 5 to 10 times every 1 to 2 hours, per physician's orders.	
___	___	___	6. Wash hands.	

Procedure Checklists to Accompany Craven/Hirnle's Fundamentals of Nursing: Human Health and Function, third edition.

Name _____ Date _____

Unit _____ Position _____

Instructor/Evaluator _____ Position _____

Excellent	Satisfactory	Needs Practice	*Procedure 33-4* **Monitoring Peak Flow**	COMMENTS
▼	▼	▼	**Goal:** To measure peak expiratory flow rate (PEFR) to assess respiratory function especially for clients with asthma.	
___	___	___	1. Explain purpose of peak flow monitoring to the client and family.	
___	___	___	2. Place indicator at base of numbered scale. Have client stand up.	
___	___	___	3. Instruct client to take a deep breath. Place the meter in his or her mouth. Have client close lips around the mouth piece. Remind client to keep tongue out of the hole.	
___	___	___	4. Instruct client to exhale as fast and as hard as he or she can, keeping a tight fit around the mouthpiece.	
___	___	___	5. Repeat steps 2 to 4 twice more, and record the highest peak flow obtained in the three attempts.	
___	___	___	6. To determine "personal best" when beginning peak flow monitoring, obtain peak flow measurements in the morning and again in the evening over a 2-week period of good asthma control. The client should take measurements before using bronchodilators.	
___	___	___	7. Healthcare provider will calculate zones based on percentage of personal best (green 80%–100%; yellow 50%–80%; red below 50%) and give instructions for what to do in each zone.	
___	___	___	8. Encourage client to comply with twice-a-day peak flow monitoring before bronchodilator therapy and to follow heatlhcare provider's instructions for peak flows in each zone.	
___	___	___	9. Repeat Steps 2 to 5.	

Procedure Checklists to Accompany Craven/Hirnle's Fundamentals of Nursing: Human Health and Function, third edition.

Name _____ Date _____

Unit _____ Position _____

Instructor/Evaluator _____ Position _____

Procedure 33-5

Administering Oxygen by Nasal Cannula or Mask

Goal: To deliver low to moderate levels of oxygen to relieve hypoxia.

Excellent ▼	Satisfactory ▼	Needs Practice ▼		COMMENTS
___	___	___	1. Wash hands.	
___	___	___	2. Explain procedure to client. Explain that oxygen will ease dyspnea or discomfort and inform client of safety precautions associated with oxygen use. If using cannula, encourage client to breathe through nose.	
___	___	___	3. Assist client to semi- or high-Fowler's position, if tolerated.	
___	___	___	4. Insert flow meter into wall outlet. Attach oxygen tubing to nozzle on flow meter. If using high O_2 flow, attach humidifier.	
___	___	___	5. Turn on the oxygen at the prescribed rate. Check that oxygen is flowing through tubing.	
___	___	___	6. Cannula:	
___	___	___	a. Place cannula prongs into nares.	
___	___	___	b. Wrap tubing over and behind ears.	
___	___	___	c. Adjust plastic slide under chin until cannula fits snugly.	
			7. Mask:	
___	___	___	a. Place mask on face, applying from the nose and over the chin.	
___	___	___	b. Adjust metal rim over the nose and contour the mask to fit the face.	
___	___	___	c. Adjust elastic ban around head so mask fits snugly.	
___	___	___	8. Assess for proper functioning of equipment and observe client's initial response to therapy.	

Excellent ▼ Satisfactory ▼ Needs Practice ▼

Procedure 33-5

Administering Oxygen by Nasal Cannula or Mask (continued)

COMMENTS

Excellent	Satisfactory	Needs Practice		
——	——	——	9. Monitor continuous therapy by assessing for pressure areas on the skin and nares every 2 hours and rechecking flow rate every 4–8 hours.	
——	——	——	10. Document procedure and observations.	

Procedure Checklists to Accompany Craven/Hirnle's Fundamentals of Nursing: Human Health and Function, third edition.

Name _____ Date _____

Unit _____ Position _____

Instructor/Evaluator _____ Position _____

Excellent	Satisfactory	Needs Practice	

Procedure 33-6

Providing Tracheostomy Care

Goal: To maintain airway patency by removing mucus and encrusted secretions and to prevent infection or skin breakdown at stoma site.

COMMENTS

1. Wash hands and don gloves.

2. Explain procedure and purpose to client. Place in semi- to high-Fowler's position.

3. Suction tracheostomy tube. Before discarding gloves, remove soiled tracheostomy dressing, and discard with catheter inside glove:

   a. Turn suction device on and adjust pressure: infants and children, 50–75 mmHg; adults, 100–120 mmHg.

   b. Open and prepare sterile suction catheter kit.

   c. Unfold sterile cup, touching only the outside. Place on bedside table.

   d. Pour sterile saline into cup.

   e. Pick up catheter with dominant hand and attach to suction tubing without contaminating sterile hand.

   f. Place catheter end into NaCl. Test functioning of equipment by applying thumb from nondominant hand over open port to create suction.

   g. Without applying suction, gently insert catheter through tracheostomy tube and advance about 10–12 cm in adult.

   h. Apply suction by placing thumb of nondominant hand over open port. Rotate catheter with dominant hand as you withdraw the catheter. This should take 5–10 seconds.

4. Replace oxygen or humidification source and encourage client to deep-breathe as you prepare sterile supplies.

Excellent	Satisfactory	Needs Practice	
▼	▼	▼	

Procedure 33-6

Providing Tracheostomy Care (continued)

COMMENTS

___	___	___	5. Open sterile tracheostomy kit. Don sterile gloves. Pour normal saline into one basin, hydrogen peroxide into the second. Open several cotton-tipped applicators and one sterile precut tracheostomy dressing and place on sterile field. If kit does not contain twill tape, cut two 15-inch ties and set aside.
___	___	___	6. Remove oxygen or humidity source. For tracheostomy tube with inner cannula, complete Steps 8–26. For tracheostomy tube without inner cannula or plugged with a button, complete Steps 13–26.
___	___	___	7. Unlock inner cannula by turning counterclockwise. Remove inner cannula and place in basin with hydrogen peroxide.
___	___	___	8. Replace oxygen source over or near outer cannula, if needed.
___	___	___	9. Clean lumen and sides of inner cannula using pipe cleaners or sterile brush.
___	___	___	10. Rinse inner cannula thoroughly by agitating in normal saline for several seconds.
___	___	___	11. Remove oxygen source and replace inner cannula into outer cannula. "Lock" by turning clockwise until the two blue dots align. Replace oxygen or humidity source.
___	___	___	12. Clean stoma under faceplate with circular motion using hydrogen peroxide-soaked cotton-tipped applicators. Cleanse dried secretions from all exposed outer cannula surfaces.
___	___	___	13. Remove foaming secretions using normal saline-soaked cotton-tipped applicators.
___	___	___	14. Pat moist surfaces dry with 4 × 4 inch gauze.
___	___	___	15. Place dry, sterile, precut tracheostomy dressing around tracheostomy stoma and under faceplate. Does not use cut 4 × 4 inch gauze.
___	___	___	16. If tracheostomy ties are to be changed, have assistant don a sterile glove to hold the tracheostomy tube in place.
___	___	___	17. Cut a 1/2 inch slit approximately 1 inch from one end of both clean tracheostomy ties.
___	___	___	18. Remove and discard soiled tracheostomy ties.

96

Excellent	Satisfactory	Needs Practice	

Procedure 33-6

Providing Tracheostomy Care (continued)

COMMENTS

___ ___ ___			19. Thread the slit end of one clean tie through the one eyelet of the faceplate. Thread the other end of the tie through the slit and pull it taut against the faceplate.
___ ___ ___			20. Repeat Step 20 with the second tie.
___ ___ ___			21. Bring both ties together at one side of client's neck. Assess that ties are only tight enough to allow one finger between tie and neck. Use two square knots to secure the ties. Trim excess tie length.
___ ___ ___			22. Remove gloves and discard disposable equipment. Label, date, and store reusable supplies.
___ ___ ___			23. Assist client to comfortable position and offer oral hygiene.
___ ___ ___			24. Wash hands.
___ ___ ___			25. Document procedure and observations.

Procedure Checklists to Accompany Craven/Hirnle's Fundamentals of Nursing: Human Health and Function, third edition.

Name _____ Date _____

Unit _____ Position _____

Instructor/Evaluator _____ Position _____

Excellent	Satisfactory	Needs Practice	*Procedure 33-7* **Suctioning Secretions from Airways**	
▼	▼	▼	**Goal:** To maintain patient airway by removing secretions.	**COMMENTS**
——	——	——	1. Wash hands.	
——	——	——	2. Explain procedure and purpose to client.	
——	——	——	3a. Position the client with an intact gag reflex in semi-Fowler's position.	
——	——	——	3b. Position the unconscious client in side-lying position facing you.	
——	——	——	4. Turn suction device on and adjust pressure: infants and children, 50–75 mmHg; adults, 100–120 mmHg.	
——	——	——	5. Open and prepare sterile suction catheter kit:	
——	——	——	a. Unfold sterile cup, touching only the outside. Place on bedside table.	
——	——	——	b. Pour sterile saline into cup.	
——	——	——	6. Preoxygenate client with 100% oxygen. Hyperinflate with manual resuscitation bag.	
——	——	——	7. Don sterile gloves. If kit supplies only one glove, place on dominant hand.	
——	——	——	8. Pick up catheter with dominant hand. Pick up connecting tubing with nondominant hand. Attach catheter to tubing without contaminating sterile hand.	
——	——	——	9. Place catheter end into cup of saline. Test functioning of equipment by applying thumb from nondominant hand over open port to create suction. Return catheter to sterile field.	
——	——	——	10. Insert catheter into trachea through nostril, nasal trumpet, or artificial airway during inspiration.	
——	——	——	11. Advance catheter until resistance is felt. Retract catheter one cm before applying suction.	

Excellent ▼	Satisfactory ▼	Needs Practice ▼	*Procedure 33-7* **Suctioning Secretions from Airways (continued)**	COMMENTS
——	——	——	12. Apply suction by placing thumb of nondominant hand over open port. Rotate catheter with your dominant hand as you withdraw the catheter. This should take 5–10 seconds.	
——	——	——	13. Hyperoxygenate and hyperinflate using manual resuscitation bag for a full minute between subsequent suction passes. Encourage deep breathing.	
——	——	——	14. Rinse catheter thoroughly with saline.	
——	——	——	15. Repeat Steps 10–14 until airway is clear.	
——	——	——	16. Without applying suction, insert the catheter gently along one side of the mouth. Advance to the oropharynx.	
——	——	——	17. Apply suction for 5–10 seconds as you rotate and withdraw the catheter. Be sure to remove secretions that pool beneath the tongue and in the vestibule of the mouth.	
——	——	——	18. Allow 1–2 minutes between passes for the client to ventilate. Encourage deep breathing. Replace oxygen if applicable.	
——	——	——	19. Repeat Steps 16 and 17 as necessary to clear oropharynx.	
——	——	——	20. Rinse catheter and tubing by suctioning saline through the catheter.	
——	——	——	21. Remove gloves by holding catheter with dominant hand and pulling glove off inside-out. Catheter will remain coiled inside glove. Pull other glove off inside-out. Dispose of in trash receptacle.	
——	——	——	22. Turn off suction device.	
——	——	——	23. Assist client to comfortable position. Offer assistance with oral and nasal hygiene. Replace oxygen delivery system if used.	
——	——	——	24. Dispose of disposable supplies.	
——	——	——	25. Wash hands.	
——	——	——	26. Ensure that sterile suction kit is available at head of bed.	
——	——	——	27. Document procedure and observations.	

Procedure Checklists to Accompany Craven/Hirnle's Fundamentals of Nursing: Human Health and Function, third edition.

Name _____ Date _____

Unit _____ Position _____

Instructor/Evaluator _____ Position _____

Excellent	Satisfactory	Needs Practice	Procedure 33-8 **Managing an Obstructed Airway (Heimlich Maneuver)**	COMMENTS
▼	▼	▼	**Goal:** To remove foreign body from obstructing the airway in order to prevent anoxia and cardiopulmonary arrest.	
			Conscious Child or Adult	
___	___	___	1. Client is standing or sitting.	
___	___	___	2. Stand behind client.	
___	___	___	3. Wrap your arms around client's waist.	
___	___	___	4. Make a fist with one hand. Place thumb side of fist against client's abdomen, above naval but below the xiphoid process.	
___	___	___	5. Grasp fist with other hand.	
___	___	___	6. Press fist into abdomen with a quick, upward thrust.	
___	___	___	7. Repeat distinct, separate thrusts until foreign body is expelled or client becomes unconscious.	
			Unconcious Client (Heimlich Maneuver, Abdominal Thrust)	
___	___	___	1. Client is lying on ground.	
___	___	___	2. Turn client on back and call for help.	
___	___	___	3. Finger sweep:	
___	___	___	a. Use tongue-jaw lift to open mouth.	
___	___	___	b. Insert index finger inside cheek and sweep to base of tongue. Use hooking motion if possible to dislodge and remove foreign body. Avoid finger sweeps in infants and children because you can easily push foreign body farther into airway. Remove only if clearly visible and easy to reach.	
___	___	___	4. Straddle client's thighs or kneel to the side of thighs.	

Excellent	Satisfactory	Needs Practice	
▼	▼	▼	

Procedure 33-8

Managing an Obstructed Airway (Heimlich Maneuver) (continued)

COMMENTS

Excellent	Satisfactory	Needs Practice	
____	____	____	5. Place heel of one hand on epigastric area, midline above the navel but below the xiphoid process.
____	____	____	6. Place second hand on top of first hand.
____	____	____	7. Press heel of hand into abdomen with a quick, upward thrust.
____	____	____	8. Repeat abdominal thrusts 6–10 times.
____	____	____	9. If airway is still obstructed, attempt to ventilate using mouth-to-mouth respiration and head tilt/chin lift.
____	____	____	10. Repeat Steps 5–8 until successful.

Children Younger than One Year of Age (Back Blows and Chest Thrusts)

Excellent	Satisfactory	Needs Practice	
____	____	____	1. Straddle infant over your arm with head lower than trunk.
____	____	____	2. Support head by holding jaw firmly in your hand.
____	____	____	3. Rest your forearm on your thigh and deliver four back blows with the heel of your hand between the infant's scapulae.
____	____	____	4. Place free hand on infant's back and support neck while turning to supine position.
____	____	____	5. Place two fingers over sternum in same location as for external chest compression (one finger width below nipple line).
____	____	____	6. Administer four chest thrusts.
____	____	____	7. Repeat Steps 1–6 until airway is not obstructed.

Children Older than One Year of Age

Excellent	Satisfactory	Needs Practice	
____	____	____	1. Perform Heimlich maneuver with child standing, sitting, or lying as for adult, but more gently.
____	____	____	2. You may need to kneel behind child or have child stand on a table.
____	____	____	3. Prevent foreign body airway obstruction in infants and children by teaching parents or caregivers to:
____	____	____	a. Restrict children from walking, running, or playing with food or foreign objects in their mouths.
____	____	____	b. Keep small objects (e.g., marbles, beads, beans) away from children younger than 3 years of age.

Excellent ▼	Satisfactory ▼	Needs Practice ▼	*Procedure 33-8* # Managing an Obstructed Airway (Heimlich Maneuver) (continued)
			COMMENTS

Excellent	Satisfactory	Needs Practice	
___	___	___	c. Avoid feeding popcorn and peanuts to children younger than 3 years of age, and cut other foods into small pieces.
___	___	___	4. Instruct parents and caregivers in the management of foreign body airway obstruction.
			Pregnant Women or Very Obese Adults (Chest Thrusts)
___	___	___	1. Stand behind client.
___	___	___	2. Bring your arms under client's armpits and around chest.
___	___	___	3. Make a fist and place thumb side against middle of sternum.
___	___	___	4. Grasp fist with other hand and deliver a quick, backward thrust.
___	___	___	5. Repeat thrusts until airway is cleared.
___	___	___	6. Chest thrusts may be performed with client supine and hands positioned with heel over lower half of sternum. Administer separate, downward thrusts until airway is clear.

Procedure Checklists to Accompany Craven/Hirnle's Fundamentals of Nursing: Human Health and Function, third edition.

Name _____   Date _____

Unit _____   Position _____

Instructor/Evaluator _____   Position _____

Excellent	Satisfactory	Needs Practice	
▼	▼	▼	**Procedure 34-1** **Applying Antiembolic Stockings** **Goal:** To supplement the action of muscle contraction and aid venous return from lower extremities.	**COMMENTS**
___	___	___	1. Gather equipment.	
___	___	___	2. Wash hands.	
___	___	___	3. Explain procedure and purpose to client.	
___	___	___	4. Position client in supine position for one-half hour before applying stockings.	
___	___	___	5. Provide for client's privacy.	
___	___	___	6. Measure for proper fit prior to first application. Measure length (heel to groin) and width (calf and thigh). Compare to manufacturer's printed material to ensure proper fit.	
___	___	___	7. Turn stocking inside out, tucking foot inside.	
___	___	___	8. Ease the foot section over the client's toe and heel, adjusting as necessary for proper, smooth fit.	
___	___	___	9. Gently pull the stocking over the leg, removing all wrinkles. Baby powder or talc sprinkled over foot and leg may make stocking application easier.	
___	___	___	10. Assess toes for circulation and warmth. Check area at top of stocking for binding.	
___	___	___	11. Remove antiembolic stockings at least twice daily.	

Procedure Checklists to Accompany Craven/Hirnle's Fundamentals of Nursing: Human Health and Function, third edition.

Name _____ Date _____

Unit _____ Position _____

Instructor/Evaluator _____ Position _____

Procedure 34-2
Applying Sequential Compression Device (SCD)

Goal: To promote venous return from legs to decrease the risk of deep vein thrombosis and pulmonary embolism.

Excellent	Satisfactory	Needs Practice		COMMENTS
___	___	___	1. Gather equipment.	
___	___	___	2. Wash hands.	
___	___	___	3. Explain procedure and purpose to client.	
___	___	___	4. Provide for client privacy.	
___	___	___	5. Measure leg to ensure proper sleeve sizing. Knee length: one size fits all; thigh length—measure length of leg from ankle to popliteal fossa. Measure circumference of thigh at gluteal fold: Extra small—circumference 22 inches; length 16 inches Regular—circumference 29 inches; length 16 inches Extra large—circumference 35 inches; length 16 inches	
___	___	___	6. Apply antiembolism stockings. Ensure that there are no wrinkles or folds (see Procedure 34-1). Use stockinette or ace wraps if unable to fit client with antiembolism stockings.	
___	___	___	7. Place client in supine position.	
___	___	___	8. Place a plastic sleeve under each leg so the opening is at the knee.	
___	___	___	9. Fold outer section of the sleeve over the inner portion, and secure with Velcro tabs. Check sleeve fit. Two fingers should fit between the sleeve and leg.	
___	___	___	10. Connect tubing to control unit. Align arrows on tubing and controller to make adequate connection. Turn on machine.	

Excellent	Satisfactory	Needs Practice	

Procedure 34-2

Applying Sequential Compression Device (SCD) (continued)

COMMENTS

Excellent	Satisfactory	Needs Practice		
___	___	___	11. Adjust control unit settings as necessary. Unit control is preset with sleeve cooling in "Off" position and audible alarm in "On" position. Sleeve cooling should be "On" at all times except during surgery. Ankle pressure should be set at 35–55 mmHg.	
___	___	___	12. Recheck control unit settings whenever unit has been turned off.	
___	___	___	13. Respond to and promptly correct all "Fault" indicator alarms.	
___	___	___	14. Document time and date of application. If SCD is applied to only one leg, document reason.	
___	___	___	15. Assess and document skin integrity every 8 hours.	
___	___	___	16. Remove sleeves and notify physician if client experiences tingling, numbness, or leg pain.	

Procedure Checklists to Accompany Craven/Hirnle's Fundamentals of Nursing: Human Health and Function, third edition.

Name _____ Date _____

Unit _____ Position _____

Instructor/Evaluator _____ Position _____

Excellent	Satisfactory	Needs Practice	*Procedure 34-3* **Administering Cardiopulmonary Resuscitation (CPR)**	COMMENTS
▼	▼	▼	**Goal:** To restore cardiopulmonary functioning.	
			One Rescuer—Adult Client	
___	___	___	1. Ask, "Are you okay?" Assess to determine responsiveness. Shake gently.	
___	___	___	2. Call for help.	
___	___	___	3. Turn client onto back while supporting head and neck. Place a cardiac board under back or place client on floor.	
___	___	___	4. Open the airway:	
___	___	___	a. Use a head tilt/chin lift maneuver.	
___	___	___	b. Use modified jaw thrust if a neck injury is suspected.	
___	___	___	5. Place your ear over client's mouth, and observe the chest for rising with respiration. *Listen, look, and feel* for breathing for 3–5 seconds.	
___	___	___	6. Pinch the client's nostrils with thumb and index finger of hand holding the forehead.	
___	___	___	7. Take a deep breath and place your mouth around the client's mouth with a tight seal. If client wears dentures, they should remain in place.	
___	___	___	8. Ventilate two full breaths. Each breath takes 1.5–2 seconds to deliver. Pause between breaths to allow for lung deflation and to take another deep breath.	
___	___	___	9. Assess for carotid pulse for 5–10 seconds on the side next to which you are kneeling. Maintain head tilt with other hand.	
___	___	___	10. If client is pulseless, start chest compressions.	

Procedure 34-3

Administering Cardiopulmonary Resuscitation (CPR) (continued)

Excellent ▼	Satisfactory ▼	Needs Practice ▼		COMMENTS
___	___	___	11. With hand nearest client's legs, place middle and index fingers on lower ridge of ribs and move fingers up along ribs to costal-sternal notch (in center of lower chest).	
___	___	___	12. Place middle finger on this notch and index finger next to the middle finger on the lower end of the notch.	
___	___	___	13. Place heel of other hand along the lower half of the sternum, next to the index finger.	
___	___	___	14. Remove first hand from the notch and place heel of that hand parallel over the hand on the chest. Interlock fingers, keeping them off client's chest.	
___	___	___	15. Keeping your hands on sternum, extend your arms, locking the elbows, with your shoulders directly over the client's chest.	
___	___	___	16. Press down on chest, depressing sternum 1.5–2 inches.	
___	___	___	17. Completely release compression while maintaining your hand position. Repeat in a smooth rhythm 80–100 times/minute.	
___	___	___	18. Ventilate with two full breaths after every 15 chest compressions.	
___	___	___	19. Repeat four cycles of 15 chest compressions and two ventilations.	
___	___	___	20. Reassess for carotid pulse. If client is pulseless, continue CPR. Reassess for carotid pulse every few minutes without interrupting CPR for longer than 7 seconds.	

Two Rescuers—Adult Client

Excellent	Satisfactory	Needs Practice		COMMENTS
___	___	___	1. When second rescuer arrives, the first rescuer stops CPR after completing two ventilations and assesses for a carotid pulse for 5 seconds.	
___	___	___	2. Second rescuer moves into chest compression position.	
___	___	___	3. If pulselessness continues, the first rescuer states "No pulse" and delivers one ventilation.	
___	___	___	4. Second rescuer begins chest compression while counting out loud, "One and two and three and four and five and." The compression rate is 80–100/minute.	

Procedure 34-3
Administering Cardiopulmonary Resuscitation (CPR) (continued)

Excellent ▼ **Satisfactory** ▼ **Needs Practice** ▼

COMMENTS

___ ___ ___ 5. First rescuer gives one full ventilation after every five chest compressions. First rescuer also assesses carotid pulse during chest compresions to evaluate effectiveness.

___ ___ ___ 6. If second rescuer wishes to change positions, he or she states, "Change, one and two and three and four and five and."

___ ___ ___ 7. First rescuer delivers the ventilation then moves into the chest compression position.

___ ___ ___ 8. Second rescuer moves to the ventilator position and assesses for a carotid pulse for 5 seconds. If pulseless, resume CPR. Do not interrupt CPR for more than 7 seconds.

One Rescuer CPR—Infant and Child

___ ___ ___ 1. Assess unresponsiveness.

___ ___ ___ 2. Call for help.

___ ___ ___ 3. Place child on hard surface. Provide basic life support for one full minute before activating emergency medical system.

___ ___ ___ 4. Open airway using head tilt/chin lift. Avoid overextension of head in infants.

___ ___ ___ 5. Place your ear over child's mouth, and observe chest for rise. Listen, look, and feel for breathing. Perform Heimlich maneuver if airway obstruction is suspected.

___ ___ ___ 6. If breathlessness is determined, seal mouth and nose and ventilate twice (1–1.5 seconds for each breath). Observe for chest rise.

___ ___ ___ 7. Assess pulselessness by palpating for carotid artery on near side in children older than one year, in infants younger than one year, assess brachial or femoral pulse for 5 seconds.

___ ___ ___ 8. Begin chest compression if pulseless:

___ ___ ___ a. For infant up to one year:

___ ___ ___ 1. Visualize an imaginary line between the infant's nipples.

___ ___ ___ 2. Place index finger on sternum just below imaginary line.

Procedure 34-3

Administering Cardiopulmonary Resuscitation (CPR) (continued)

Excellent ▼	Satisfactory ▼	Needs Practice ▼		COMMENTS
___	___	___	3. Place middle and fourth finger on sternum next to index finger for chest compressions.	
___	___	___	b. For child 1–8 years of age:	
___	___	___	1. Placement of hand on sternum is same as for adult CPR. Use heel of one hand to compress sternum 1–1.5 inches 80–100 times/minute.	
___	___	___	2. Continue chest compessions, and ventilate at the rate of one breath to five compressions.	
___	___	___	3. Continue CPR as for an adult.	

Procedure Checklists to Accompany Craven/Hirnle's Fundamentals of Nursing: Human Health and Function, third edition.

Name _____ Date _____

Unit _____ Position _____

Instructor/Evaluator _____ Position _____

Procedure 36-1

Measuring Blood Glucose by Skin Puncture

Goal: To monitor blood glucose levels for clients who are at risk for hypoglycemia or hyperglycemia.

Excellent	Satisfactory	Needs Practice		COMMENTS
▼	▼	▼		
___	___	___	1. Have client wash hands with soap and warm water.	
___	___	___	2. Position client comfortably.	
___	___	___	3. Remove reagent strip from the container and handle according to the manufacturer's instructions.	
___	___	___	4. Place reagent strip with test pad up on a dry surface.	
___	___	___	5. Choose the finger to be punctured, massage gently, and hold in a dependent position.	
___	___	___	6. Wipe the puncture site with alcohol (or a povidone-iodine swab). Allow site to dry completely.	
___	___	___	7. Don gloves.	
___	___	___	8. Remove the cover of the lancet or autolet. Place the autolet against the side of the finger and push the release button. If using a lancet, hold it perpendicular to the side and pierce the site quickly.	
___	___	___	9. Wipe the initial drop of blood with a cotton ball.	
___	___	___	10. Squeeze the puncture gently or massage the skin toward the site to obtain a large drip of blood. Hold reagent strip next to drop of blood and allow blood to cover the test pad completely. Do not smear the blood. In some meters, bring the finger to the test site on the meter and allow blood to drop onto appropriate area.	
___	___	___	11. Start timing (usually less than 60 seconds) using the glucose meter, or a watch if the meter is not available.	
___	___	___	12. Following manufacturer's instructions, wipe the blood from the test pad with a cotton ball after the specified period of time.	

Procedure 36-1

Measuring Blood Glucose
by Skin Puncture (continued)

Excellent	Satisfactory	Needs Practice		COMMENTS
___	___	___	13. Place the reagent strip into the glucose meter. After the recommended period of time, read the results. For meters on which blood is placed directly, read the results at the designated time. If a glucose meter is not available, compare the color of the test pad with the color strip on the side of the reagent strip container.	
___	___	___	14. Turn off the glucose meter. Dispose of used equipment in the appropriate manner.	
___	___	___	15. Share test results with client and record obtained values in the client's chart.	

Procedure Checklists to Accompany Craven/Hirnle's Fundamentals of Nursing: Human Health and Function, third edition.

Name _____ Date _____

Unit _____ Position _____

Instructor/Evaluator _____ Position _____

Excellent ▼	Satisfactory ▼	Needs Practice ▼	*Procedure 36-2* **Assisting An Adult with Feeding**
			Goal: To maintain nutritional status. COMMENTS
____	____	____	1. Prepare client's environment for meal:
____	____	____	a. Remove urinals, bedpans, dressings, trash.
____	____	____	b. Ventilate or aerate room for unpleasant odors.
____	____	____	c. Clean overbed table.
____	____	____	2. Prepare client for meal:
____	____	____	a. Help client to urinate or defecate.
____	____	____	b. Help client to wash face and hands.
____	____	____	c. Assist with oral hygiene.
____	____	____	d. Help client to apply dentures, glasses, or special appliances.
____	____	____	e. Assist to upright position in bed or chair.
____	____	____	3. Wash your hands before touching meal tray.
____	____	____	4. Check client's tray against diet order.
____	____	____	5. Place tray on overbed table and move in front of client.
____	____	____	6. Prepare tray. Open cartons, remove lids, season food, cut food into bite-size pieces.
____	____	____	7. Place napkin or towel under client's chin, and cover clothing.
____	____	____	8. If client can feed self, leave and return in 10–15 minutes to determine if client is tolerating diet. (Do not leave client with overly hot liquids or food unless fully independent with feeding.)
____	____	____	9. a. If client can sit in a chair but needs help to eat, sit in chair facing client.
____	____	____	b. If client must remain in bed, nurse may stand to feed client.

Excellent ▼	Satisfactory ▼	Needs Practice ▼	

Procedure 36-2
Assisting An Adult with Feeding (continued)

COMMENTS

Excellent	Satisfactory	Needs Practice		
___	___	___	10. Allow client to choose the order in which he or she would like to eat. If client is visually impaired, identify the food on the tray.	
___	___	___	11. Warn client if food is hot or cold.	
___	___	___	12. Allow enough time between bites for adequate chewing and swallowing.	
___	___	___	13. Offer liquids as requested or between bites. Use straw or special drinking cup, if available.	
___	___	___	14. Provide conversation during meal. Choose topic of interest to client. Reorient to current events or use meal as opportunity to educate on nutrition or discharge plans. Do *not* talk to clients who are relearning swallowing techniques; they need to concentrate.	
___	___	___	15. Help client to wash hands and face, and perform oral hygiene after meal.	
___	___	___	16. Assist to comfortable position and allow rest period. If at risk for aspiration, leave head of bed elevated for 30 minutes after eating.	
___	___	___	17. Record fluids and amount of meal consumed, if ordered.	
___	___	___	18. Remove and dispose of tray.	
___	___	___	19. Wash hands.	

Procedure Checklists to Accompany Craven/Hirnle's Fundamentals of Nursing: Human Health and Function, third edition.

Name _____ Date _____

Unit _____ Position _____

Instructor/Evaluator _____ Position _____

Excellent	Satisfactory	Needs Practice	
▼	▼	▼	**Procedure 36-3** ## Administering Nutrition via Nasogastric or Gastrostomy Tube **Goal:** To provide enteral nutrition for clients who cannot swallow or who have an esophageal obstruction.

				COMMENTS
___	___	___	1. Wash hands.	
___	___	___	2. Close room door or curtains around bed.	
___	___	___	3. Explain procedure and purpose to client.	
___	___	___	4. Help client to high-Fowler's position by elevating head of bed at least 60 degrees or by assisting to chair. If high-Fowler's position is contraindicated, help client to a right side-lying position with head slightly elevated.	
___	___	___	5. Confirm placement of tube in stomach:	
___	___	___	a. Withdraw sample of stomach contents and check for low pH level.	
___	___	___	b. Attach 60 mL-irrigation syringe to tube and inject 10 mL of air while auscultating over epigastrium. Recognize that this may not be reliable index of tube placement when client has small-bore feeding tube.	
___	___	___	c. Aspirate all stomach contents and measure residual.	
___	___	___	d. If 100 mL, or more than half of last feeding, is aspirated, contact physician before proceeding with tube feeding. The feeding is usually held.	
___	___	___	e. Reinstill the aspirated gastric contents through tube into stomach.	
___	___	___	6. Prepare correct amount and strength of formula at room temperature. (Optional: Add several drops of food coloring.)	

Procedure 36-3

Administering Nutrition via Nasogastric or Gastrostomy Tube (continued)

Excellent	Satisfactory	Needs Practice	
▼	▼	▼	**COMMENTS**

Bolus of Intermittent Feeding

_____ _____ _____ 1. Remove plunger from irrigation syringe. Clamp gastric tubing and attach syringe. If using gavage bag, attach tubing to gastric tube.

_____ _____ _____ 2. Fill syringe or gavage bag with formula.

_____ _____ _____ 3. Allow feeding to flow in slowly over 10–15 minutes. If using syringe, raise and lower to adjust flow rate by gravity. Refill syringe as needed without disconnecting, avoiding air spaces in tubing. If gavage bag is used, hang bag on IV pole and adjust flow rate with clamp on tubing.

_____ _____ _____ 4. Clamp tubing just as feeding is completing. Rinse tube with 30–60 mL tap water. Do not allow air to enter tubing.

_____ _____ _____ 5. Clamp gastric tube and disconnect from syringe or gavage bag.

_____ _____ _____ 6. Have client remain in high-Fowler's or elevated side-lying position for 30–60 minutes.

Continuous Feeding

_____ _____ _____ 1. Connect gavage tubing to gastric tube.

_____ _____ _____ 2. Hang gavage bag on IV pole.

_____ _____ _____ 3. Pour in desired amount of formula according to agency policy. (Usually amount to infuse in 3 hours.)

_____ _____ _____ 4. a. Connect tubing to infusion pump.

_____ _____ _____   b. Set rate.

_____ _____ _____ 5. Check residual every 4–6 hours, according to agency policy. Then flush tubing with 30–60 mL water.

_____ _____ _____ 6. Have client remain in high-Fowler's or slightly elevated side-lying position for 30–60 minutes.

_____ _____ _____ 7. Wash any reusable equipment with soap and water. Change equipment every 24 hours or according to agency policy.

_____ _____ _____ 8. Wash hands.

_____ _____ _____ 9. Document procedure and observations.

Procedure Checklists to Accompany Craven/Hirnle's Fundamentals of Nursing: Human Health and Function, third edition.

Name _____ Date _____

Unit _____ Position _____

Instructor/Evaluator _____ Position _____

Excellent ▼	Satisfactory ▼	Needs Practice ▼	*Procedure 37-1* **Changing a Dry Sterile Dressing**

Goal: To protect wound from trauma and external contamination.　　**COMMENTS**

Excellent	Satisfactory	Needs Practice	
___	___	___	1. Close client's door or close curtains around bed. Explain procedure to client.
___	___	___	2. Position client in a comfortable position. Expose wound area only.
___	___	___	3. Wash hands.
___	___	___	4. Make a cuff on top of plastic bag and place within easy reach of dressing table.
___	___	___	5. Put on clean disposable gloves.
___	___	___	6. Remove dressing from wound and discard into plastic bag. If dressing adheres to wound, pour small amount of sterile saline on wound to loosen dressing.
___	___	___	7. Remove and dispose of gloves. Wash hands.
___	___	___	8. Set up sterile supplies:
___	___	___	a. Open sterile towel, and hold it by edges.
___	___	___	b. Place it on clean, flat surface without contaminating center of towel.
___	___	___	c. Open dressing package(s) by peeling paper down to expose dressing. Let it fall onto sterile field.
___	___	___	d. Open cleansing solution container and pour solution into sterile cup.
___	___	___	e. Open applicator packages. Set materials at side of sterile field. (Optional: Open dressing packages and suture set carefully, allowing the inside of the packaging material to serve as the sterile field.)
___	___	___	9. Don sterile gloves. Grasp applicators at nonabsorbent end and dip into cleansing solution.

Procedure 37-1

Changing a Dry Sterile Dressing (continued)

Excellent	Satisfactory	Needs Practice		COMMENTS
▼	▼	▼		
____	____	____	10. Clean drainage from least contaminated area to most contaminated area (outward toward the wound). Use each applicator once and discard it.	
____	____	____	11. Dry surrounding skin gently with gauze.	
____	____	____	12. Inspect incision for bleeding, inflammation, drainage, and healing. Note any areas of dehiscence.	
____	____	____	13. Apply sterile dressings one at a time over wound.	
____	____	____	14. Wash hands.	
____	____	____	15. Document procedure and observations.	

Procedure Checklists to Accompany Craven/Hirnle's Fundamentals of Nursing: Human Health and Function, third edition.

Name _____ Date _____

Unit _____ Position _____

Instructor/Evaluator _____ Position _____

Excellent	Satisfactory	Needs Practice	*Procedure 37-2* **Applying Saline-Moistened Dressings**	COMMENTS
▼	▼	▼	**Goal:** To promote moist wound healing.	
___	___	___	1. Prepare client and remove dressing according to Steps 1–5 of Procedure 37-1. Forceps may be used to remove soiled dressing. If dressing adheres to underlying tissues, moisten with saline to loosen. Gently remove the dressing while assessing client's discomfort level.	
___	___	___	2. Observe dressings for amount and characteristics of drainage. Note odor and color.	
___	___	___	3. Observe wound for eschar, granulation tissue, or epithelial skin buds. Measure and record wound depth, diameter, and length.	
___	___	___	4. Prepare sterile supplies. Open sterile instruments, sterile basin, solution, and dressings.	
___	___	___	5. Place fine-mesh gauze into basin, and pour the ordered solution over mesh to saturate. For large wounds, warm ordered solution to body temperature.	
___	___	___	6. Don sterile gloves.	
___	___	___	7. Cleanse or irrigate wound as prescribed or with normal saline, moving from least to most contaminated areas.	
___	___	___	8. Squeeze excess fluid from gauze dressing. Unfold and fluff out the dressing:	
___	___	___	a. Gently pack moistened gauze into the wound.	
___	___	___	b. If wound is deep, use forceps or cotton-tipped applicators to press gauze into all wound surfaces.	
___	___	___	9. Apply several dry, sterile 4 × 4s over the wet gauze.	
___	___	___	10. Place ABD pad over dry 4 × 4s.	
___	___	___	11. Dispose of sterile gloves.	
___	___	___	12. Secure dressings with tape, Kerlix gauze, or Montgomery ties.	

Excellent ▼	Satisfactory ▼	Needs Practice ▼	*Procedure 37-2* **Applying Saline-Moistened Dressings (continued)**
			COMMENTS
____	____	____	13. Assist client to a comfortable position.
____	____	____	14. Wash hands.
____	____	____	15. Document the procedure and observations.

Procedure Checklists to Accompany Craven/Hirnle's Fundamentals of Nursing: Human Health and Function, third edition.

Name _____ Date _____

Unit _____ Position _____

Instructor/Evaluator _____ Position _____

Procedure 37-3
Irrigating a Wound

Goal: To cleanse wound by removing debris and exudate.

Excellent	Satisfactory	Needs Practice		COMMENTS
___	___	___	1. Close door or curtains around bed. Explain procedure to client.	
___	___	___	2. Position client comfortably to allow irrigating solution to flow by gravity across wound and into a collection basin.	
___	___	___	3. Expose the wound area only. Place waterproof pad under client.	
___	___	___	4. Wash hands.	
___	___	___	5. Don mask, goggles, and gown, if needed.	
___	___	___	6. Remove dressing and inspect wound. See Steps 1–4 of Procedure 37-2.	
___	___	___	7. Pour warmed irrigating solution into sterile basin.	
___	___	___	8. Open irrigating syringe and place into basin with solution.	
___	___	___	9. Place second basin at distal end of wound to catch contaminated irrigating solution.	
___	___	___	10. Don sterile gloves.	
___	___	___	11. Fill irrigating syringe with solution. Holding syringe tip about 1 inch above the wound, and gently flush all areas of wound. Continue flushing until solution draining into basin is clear.	
___	___	___	12. If wound is deep, attach a latex or silicone catheter to syringe filled with irrigating solution. Gently insert catheter into wound and flush until returning solution is clear.	
___	___	___	13. Dry surrounding skin thoroughly.	
___	___	___	14. Apply sterile dressing.	
___	___	___	15. Remove and discard gloves.	

Excellemt	Satisfactory	Needs Practice	
▼	▼	▼	

Procedure 37-3

Irrigating a Wound (continued)

COMMENTS

____	____	____	16. Secure dressing with tape or Montgomery straps.
____	____	____	17. Assist client to comfortable position.
____	____	____	18. Dispose of equipment. Retain remaining bottle of sterile solution for future irrigations. Mark date and time of opening on bottle for reference. Dispose of according to agency policy.
____	____	____	19. Wash hands.
____	____	____	20. Document procedure and observations.

Procedure Checklists to Accompany Craven/Hirnle's Fundamentals of Nursing: Human Health and Function, third edition.

Name _____ Date _____

Unit _____ Position _____

Instructor/Evaluator _____ Position _____

Procedure 37-4

Maintaining a Portable (Hemovac) Wound Suction

Goal: To facilitate healing by removing drainage from the incisional area.

Excellemt	Satisfactory	Needs Practice		COMMENTS
▼	▼	▼		
___	___	___	1. Explain procedure, assist client to comfortable position, pull curtains or close door.	
___	___	___	2. Wash hands. Don clean, disposable gloves.	
___	___	___	3. Expose Hemovac tubing and container while keeping client draped.	
___	___	___	4. Examine tubing and container for patency and suction seal.	
___	___	___	5. Open drainage plug.	
___	___	___	6. Pour drainage into a calibrated receptacle without contaminating drainage spout.	
___	___	___	7. Reestablish suction by placing reservoir on firm, flat surface. With drainage plug open, compress the unit and reinsert drainage plug.	
___	___	___	8. Remove and discard gloves.	
___	___	___	9. Return client to comfortable position.	
___	___	___	10. Measure drainage, and record amount, color, and other pertinent information.	

122

Procedure Checklists to Accompany Craven/Hirnle's Fundamentals of Nursing: Human Health and Function, third edition.

Name _____ Date _____

Unit _____ Position _____

Instructor/Evaluator _____ Position _____

Excellemt	Satisfactory	Needs Practice	

Procedure 38-1

Obtaining a Wound Culture

Goal: To identify organisms colonized within a wound so antibiotics sensitive to the microorganisms can be prescribed as needed.

COMMENTS

1. Wash hands, and apply clean disposable gloves.
2. Remove soiled dressing. Observe drainage for amount, odor, and color.
3. Clear and remove exudate from around wound with antiseptic swab.

Obtaining Aerobic Culture

1. Perform Steps 1–3 above.
2. Using sterile swab from culture tube, insert swab deep into area of active drainage. Rotate swab to absorb as much drainage as possible.
3. Insert swab into culture tube, taking care not to touch the top or outside of tube.
4. Crush ampule of medium and close container securely.
5. Label each culture tube and send specimen with appropriate laboratory requisition immediately to the laboratory.

Obtaining Anaerobic Culture

1. Perform Steps 1–3 at beginning of procedure.
2. Using sterile swab from special anaerobic culture tube, insert swab deeply into draining body cavity.
3. a. Rotate swab gently and remove. Quickly place swab into inner tube of collection container.
   b. Alternative: Insert tip of syringe with needle removed into wound and aspirate 1–5 mL of exudate. Attach 21-gauge needle to syringe, expel all air, and inject exudate into inner tube of the culture container.

Procedure 38-1

Obtaining a Wound Culture (continued)

Excellemt	Satisfactory	Needs Practice		COMMENTS
▼	▼	▼		
___	___	___	4. Label each culture tube and send specimens with appropriate requisitions to the laboratory.	
___	___	___	5. Clean and apply sterile dressings to the wound, as ordered.	
___	___	___	6. Remove and discard gloves. Wash hands.	
___	___	___	7. Assist client to comfortable position.	
___	___	___	8. Document all relevant information on client's chart. Include the location the specimen was taken from and the date and time. Record the wound's consistency of drainage. Record how the client tolerated the procedure and any discomfort experienced.	

Procedure Checklists to Accompany Craven/Hirnle's Fundamentals of Nursing: Human Health and Function, third edition.

Name _____ Date _____

Unit _____ Position _____

Instructor/Evaluator _____ Position _____

Excellent ▼	Satisfactory ▼	Needs Practice ▼	
			## Procedure 39-1 ## Collecting Urine Specimens **Goal:** To obtain a noncontaminated urine specimen for routine analysis or culture and sensitivity.

COMMENTS

Sterile Specimen from an Indwelling Catheter

___	___	___	1. Explain procedure to client.
___	___	___	2. Wash hands. Put on clean disposable gloves.
___	___	___	3. Position client so that catheter is accessible.
___	___	___	4. Drain urine from tubing into collection bag. Allow fresh urine to collect in tubing by clamping or bending tubing (2 mL of urine is sufficient for a culture and sensitivity specimen; 30 mL for urinalysis).
___	___	___	5. Cleanse aspiration port of drainage tubing with alcohol or Betadine swab.
___	___	___	6. Insert needle into aspiration port. Draw urine sample into syringe by gentle aspiration. Remove needle.
___	___	___	7. Transfer urine from syringe into a sterile specimen container.
___	___	___	8. Label container. Date and time laboratory requisition. Place in plastic biohazard bag for delivery to laboratory.
___	___	___	9. Send specimen to laboratory within 15 minutes or place in specimen refrigerator. If specimen is for microbiology testing, do not refrigerate and send immediately.
___	___	___	10. Dispose all contaminated supplies. Wash hands.
___	___	___	11. Document procedure and observations.

Excellemt	Satisfactory	Needs Practice	

Procedure 39-1
Collecting Urine Specimens (continued)

COMMENTS

Self-Collecting Midstream Urine Specimen for a Woman

___ ___ ___ 1. Instruct client how to cleanse urinary meatus and obtain urine specimen:

___ ___ ___   a. (Client) Wash hands.

___ ___ ___   b. Separate labia minora and cleanse perineum with cleansing agent, starting in front of the urethral meatus, and moving swab toward the rectum.

___ ___ ___   c. Begin to urinate while continuing to hold labia apart. Allow first urine to flow into toilet.

___ ___ ___   d. Hold specimen container under the urine stream and collect sample.

___ ___ ___   e. Remove specimen container, release hand from labia, seal container tightly, and finish voiding. Wash hands.

___ ___ ___ 2. (Nurse) Put on disposable gloves to receive specimen container from the client. Dry outside of container with a paper towel.

___ ___ ___ 3. Date and time laboratory specimen. Label the container and place specimen container in biohazard bag.

___ ___ ___ 4. Send specimen to laboratory within 15 minutes or place in specimen refrigerator. If specimen is for microbiology testing, do not refrigerate and send immediately.

___ ___ ___ 5. Dispose of all contaminated supplies. Wash hands.

Self-Collecting Midstream Urine Specimen for a Man

___ ___ ___ 1. Instruct client how to cleanse urinary meatus and obtain urine specimen:

___ ___ ___   a. (Client) Wash hands.

___ ___ ___   b. Cleanse end of penis with cleansing agent. If man is not circumcised, instruct him to retract foreskin to expose urinary meatus before cleansing and throughout specimen collection.

___ ___ ___   c. Begin to urinate, allowing urine to flow into toilet.

___ ___ ___   d. Pass specimen container into urine stream and collect sample.

___ ___ ___   e. Remove container, seal tightly, and finish voiding.

___ ___ ___ 2. Follow Steps 2–5 above.

Excellent	Satisfactory	Needs Practice	
▼	▼	▼	*Procedure 39-1* # Collecting Urine Specimens (continued) **COMMENTS**

Collecting a Specimen from a Child without Urinary Control

___	___	___	1. If parents are present, explain procedure to them.
___	___	___	2. Position child gently on back. Put on disposable gloves. Remove diaper.
___	___	___	3. Clean perineal-genital area gently with soap and water, followed by antiseptic.
___	___	___	4. For a girl: Separate labia and cleanse from front of urethral meatus toward rectum. Rinse with water and dry with cotton balls.
___	___	___	5. For a boy: Cleanse penis and scrotum. If uncircumcised, retract foreskin and cleanse. Rinse with water and dry with gauze or cotton balls.
___	___	___	6. Remove paper backing from adhesive of collection bag.
___	___	___	7. Spread child's legs apart widely.
___	___	___	8. Apply collection bag over child's perineum, covering penis and scrotum on boy, and urinary meatus and vagina on girl. Press adhesive to secure, starting at perineum and working outward.
___	___	___	9. Place a diaper on child loosely.
___	___	___	10. Remove gloves and wash hands.
___	___	___	11. Check the collector for urine every 15 minutes.
___	___	___	12. When urine specimen is obtained, glove again, and gently remove collection bag from skin and empty urine into specimen container.
___	___	___	13. Tighten lid and cleanse outside of container if contaminated with urine and place in biohazard bag for transfer to laboratory.
___	___	___	14. Label the container. Date and time laboratory requisition.
___	___	___	15. Send specimen to laboratory within 15 minutes or place in specimen refrigerator. If specimen is for microbiology testing, do not refrigerate and send immediately.
___	___	___	16. Dispose of all contaminated supplies. Wash hands.
___	___	___	17. Document that specimen was collected and sent.

Procedure Checklists to Accompany Craven/Hirnle's Fundamentals of Nursing: Human Health and Function, third edition.

Name _____ Date _____

Unit _____ Position _____

Instructor/Evaluator _____ Position _____

Excellent	Satisfactory	Needs Practice	
▼	▼	▼	

Procedure 39-2

Applying a Condom Catheter

Goal: To provide a means of collecting urine and controlling incontinence without the risk of infection that an indwelling urinary catheter imposes.

COMMENTS

___	___	___	1. Close room door or bedside curtain. Explain procedure to client.
___	___	___	2. Wash hands.
___	___	___	3. Assist client to supine position with genitalia exposed.
___	___	___	4. Put on disposable gloves. Wash client's genitals with soap and water. Towel dry.
___	___	___	5. Trim or shave excess pubic hair from base of penis, if necessary.
___	___	___	6. Apply thin film of skin protector on penis shaft. Allow to dry for 30 seconds.
___	___	___	7. Peel paper backing from both sides of adhesive line and wrap spirally around penis shaft.
___	___	___	8. Place funnel end of pre-rolled condom against glans of penis. Unroll sheath the length of the penis, over the adhesive liner.
___	___	___	9. Attach funnel end of condom to collection system. Secure system below level of condom, avoiding kinks or loops in tubing.
___	___	___	10. Discard used supplies. Remove and discard gloves. Wash hands.
___	___	___	11. Observe penis 15–30 minutes after application of condom for swelling or changes in skin color. (If too tight, remove and reapply larger size.)
___	___	___	12. Document procedure and observations.

Procedure Checklists to Accompany Craven/Hirnle's Fundamentals of Nursing: Human Health and Function, third edition.

Name _____ Date _____

Unit _____ Position _____

Instructor/Evaluator _____ Position _____

Excellemt	Satisfactory	Needs Practice	
▼	▼	▼	**Procedure 39-3** **Inserting a Straight or Indwelling Catheter** **Goal:** To monitor urinary function, relieve bladder distension, obtain sterile urine specimen, or to provide a means for irrigating the bladder. **COMMENTS**
____	____	____	1. Explain procedure and rationale to client.
____	____	____	2. Provide client with opportunity to perform personal perineal/penile hygiene. Assist client as necessary.
____	____	____	3. Wash your hands.
			Inserting Catheter for a Woman
____	____	____	1. Position in dorsal recumbent position. Externally rotate thighs. Side-lying is alternate position.
____	____	____	2. Set up light source.
____	____	____	3. Open catheterization tray.
____	____	____	4. Slide sterile drape under client's buttocks, grasping corners of drape. Ask client to lift hips so drape can be positioned.
____	____	____	5. Don sterile gloves.
____	____	____	6. Open sterile lubricant and lubricate catheter tip. Open cleansing solution and pour over half of the sterile cotton balls. Open sterile specimen container. Inflate balloon with prefilled syringe to check for defective balloon. Aspirate fluid back into syringe and leave attached.
____	____	____	7. Place nondominant hand on labia minora and gently spread to expose urinary meatus. Visualize exact location of meatus. During cleansing and catheter insertion, do not allow labia to close over meatus until after catheter is inserted.
____	____	____	8. Using sterile hand, pick up antiseptic solution saturated cotton ball with sterile forceps.
____	____	____	9. Cleanse urinary meatus with one downward stroke. Discard cotton ball. Repeat this step three or four times.
____	____	____	10. Use forceps and dry cotton balls to absorb excess antiseptic solution.

Procedure 39-3

Inserting a Straight or Indwelling Catheter (continued)

Excellemt ▼	Satisfactory ▼	Needs Practice ▼		COMMENTS
——	——	——	11. Place distal catheter end into sterile basin. With sterile hand, pick up catheter approximately 3 inches from tip and dip into sterile lubricant. Place distal catheter end into sterile basin.	
——	——	——	12. Gently insert catheter into urethra approximately 2 inches until urine begins to drain. If no urine appears, have client cough, or reposition catheter by rotating. Have client take slow, deep breaths during catheter insertion.	
——	——	——	13. Insert catheter an additional one inch or 2.5 cm. If catheter enters vagina by mistake, leave it there as a landmark. Insert second catheter into meatus.	
——	——	——	14. Obtain urine specimen in sterile container, if ordered.	
——	——	——	15. If using straight catheter, allow bladder to empty, then remove straight catheter.	
——	——	——	16. If using indwelling catheter, inflate the retention balloon with the prefilled syringe. Check to assure placement by gently pulling on catheter.	
——	——	——	17. Connect distal end of catheter to drainage bag. (May prefer to connect prior to catheter insertion.)	
——	——	——	18. Tape catheter securely with one-inch tape to inner thigh with enough give so it will not pull when moving the legs.	
——	——	——	19. Attach drainage bag to bed frame, assuring that tubing does not fall into dependent loops or that side rails do not interfere with drainage system.	
——	——	——	20. Remove gloves. Wash hands.	
——	——	——	21. Record time procedure was completed, size of catheter inserted, amount and color of urine, and any adverse client responses.	

Inserting Catheter for a Man

Excellemt	Satisfactory	Needs Practice		COMMENTS
——	——	——	1. Position client in supine position with only genitalia exposed.	
——	——	——	2. Drape legs to mid-thigh with bath blanket or sheet.	
——	——	——	3. Open catheterization tray.	

Excellent	Satisfactory	Needs Practice	
▼	▼	▼	**Procedure 39-3** # Inserting a Straight or Indwelling Catheter (continued) COMMENTS
____	____	____	4. Put on sterile gloves. Open sterile lubricant and lubricate catheter tip. Open cleansing solution and pour over half of the sterile cotton balls. Open sterile specimen container. Inflate balloon with prefilled syringe to check for defective balloon. Aspirate fluid back into syringe and leave attached.
____	____	____	5. Place the fenestrated drape over the client's genitalia.
____	____	____	6. With nondominant hand, hold penis at a 90-degree angle to his body. If client is not circumcised, pull back foreskin with this hand to visualize the urethral meatus.
____	____	____	7. Using the sterile hand, pick up antiseptic solution-soaked cotton ball with sterile forceps.
____	____	____	8. Cleanse the urinary meatus with one downward stroke or use a circular motion from meatus to base of penis. Discard cotton ball. Repeat this step at least three to four times.
____	____	____	9. Use forceps to pick up one dry cotton ball to dry the meatus.
____	____	____	10. With sterile hand, pick up the catheter approximately 3 inches from the tip and lubricate catheter generously. Place distal catheter end into sterile basin.
____	____	____	11. Gently insert catheter into urethra (approximately 8 inches) until urine begins to drain.
____	____	____	12. Insert catheter an additional one inch, or 2.5 cm.
____	____	____	13. If using an indwelling catheter, inflate the retention balloon with the prefilled syringe.
____	____	____	14. Check for placement by gently pulling on catheter.
____	____	____	15. Connect distal end of catheter to drainage bag if necessary.
____	____	____	16. Tape catheter securely with one-inch tap to the abdomen.
____	____	____	17. In the uncircumcised male, gently replace the foreskin over the glans.
____	____	____	18. Attach drainage bag to bed frame, coiling tubing to ensure that tubing does not fall into dependent loops.
____	____	____	19. Wash hands.

Excellemt

Satisfactory

Needs Practice

Excellemt	Satisfactory	Needs Practice	
▼	▼	▼	

Procedure 39-3

Inserting a Straight or Indwelling Catheter (continued)

COMMENTS

___	___	___	20. Record time procedure was completed, size of catheter, amount and color of urine, and any adverse client responses.

Removing an Indwelling Catheter

___	___	___	1. Wash hands.
___	___	___	2. Don clean, disposable gloves.
___	___	___	3. Clamp catheter (optional).
___	___	___	4. Insert hub of syringe into balloon inflation tube of catheter and draw out all liquid.
___	___	___	5. Ask client to breathe in and out deeply. Pinch gently and remove catheter as client exhales.
___	___	___	6. Assist client to cleanse and dry genitals.
___	___	___	7. Measure and document urine in drainage bag and time of catheter removal.
___	___	___	8. Wash hands.

Procedure Checklists to Accompany Craven/Hirnle's Fundamentals of Nursing: Human Health and Function, third edition.

Name _____ Date _____

Unit _____ Position _____

Instructor/Evaluator _____ Position _____

Excellemt	Satisfactory	Needs Practice	
▼	▼	▼	*Procedure 40-1* **Assessing Stool for Occult Blood** **Goal:** To screen clients who have or are at risk for gastrointestinal bleeding.

COMMENTS

____	____	____	1. Ask client to void before collecting stool specimen.
____	____	____	2. Assist client onto bedpan, commode, or to bathroom. Provide privacy and leave call bell within reach.
____	____	____	3. When client has passed stool and is clean and comfortable, don disposable gloves and obtain small amount of stool with tongue blade or wooden applicator.

Hemoccult Slide Test

____	____	____	1. Open flap of slide and apply a very thin smear of stool taken from center of the specimen onto first window.
____	____	____	2. Using second applicator, obtain a second sample from a different area of stool. Smear thinly on second window of slide.
____	____	____	3. Close slide cover. Open flap on reverse side and apply two drops of hemoccult developing solution onto each window.
____	____	____	4. Wait 30–60 seconds. Read test results.

Test with Hematest Tablets

____	____	____	1. Apply small smear of stool onto guaiac filter paper.
____	____	____	2. Place Hematest tablet on stool sample.
____	____	____	3. Apply two to three drips of water onto Hematest tablet. Hold paper so water runs onto it.
____	____	____	4. Read test results within 2 minutes by observing color of guaiac paper.
____	____	____	5. Remove gloves, wash hands, and document findings.

Procedure Checklists to Accompany Craven/Hirnle's Fundamentals of Nursing: Human Health and Function, third edition.

Name _____ Date _____

Unit _____ Position _____

Instructor/Evaluator _____ Position _____

Procedure 40-2

Administering an Enema

Goal: To relieve constipation, gas or fecal impaction, and to prepare bowel for diagnostic examinations by cleansing.

Excellemt	Satisfactory	Needs Practice		COMMENTS
▼	▼	▼		
___	___	___	1. Assemble needed equipment in one place, then provide privacy by closing curtains or room door.	
___	___	___	2. Have client lie on left side (Sim's position) with right knee flexed.	
___	___	___	3. Put on disposable gloves.	
___	___	___	4. Place waterproof towel under client's buttocks.	
___	___	___	5. Cover client with bath blanket, exposing only the rectum.	
			Large-Volume Enema	
___	___	___	1. See Steps 1–5 above.	
___	___	___	2. Fill enema bag with 750–1000 mL lukewarm solution at 105°–110°F; for a child, 500 mL or less at 100°F. Check temperature of solution with bath thermometer or by pouring some over inner wrist.	
___	___	___	3. Open clamp on tubing and flush solution to remove air. Reclamp tubing.	
___	___	___	4. Lubricate 2–3 inches of tip of rectal tube with water-soluble lubricant.	
___	___	___	5. Separate buttocks to visualize anus. Observe for external hemorrhoids. Ask client to take slow, deep breath, and gently insert rectal tube directing tip toward the umbilicus (adult, 3–4 inches).	
___	___	___	6. Continue holding tube in rectum. With other hand, open clamp and allow solution to slowly enter client. Raise container 18 inches above the anus, allowing solution to flow in slowly over a period of 5–10 minutes. If client complains of cramping or pain, have client breathe deeply and lower bag until sensation stops.	
___	___	___	7. Reclamp tubing when desired amount of solution has infused.	

Procedure 40-2

Administering an Enema (continued)

Excellemt	Satisfactory	Needs Practice		COMMENTS
▼	▼	▼		
____	____	____	8. Remove tube gently and have client squeeze buttocks together firmly for several minutes.	
____	____	____	9. Have client retain solution as long as possible.	
____	____	____	10. Assist client to bathroom, commode, or bedpan. Place call bell within reach. Provide privacy until all solution has been expelled.	
____	____	____	11. Visually inspect character of the feces and solution.	
____	____	____	12. Assist client into comfortable position.	
____	____	____	13. Assist with cleansing of client as needed. Provide materials for client to wash hands. Open windows or provide air freshener if needed. Clean and dispose of equipment as necessary. Remove gloves and wash your hands.	
____	____	____	14. Document procedure and observations.	

Small-Volume Enema

____	____	____	1. See Steps 1–5 at beginning of procedure.	
____	____	____	2. Remove protective cap from prelubricated catheter tip.	
____	____	____	3. Separate the buttocks to visualize the anus. Observe for hemorrhoids and gently insert rectal tip into rectum. Advance 3–4 inches in an adult, directing the tip toward the umbilicus.	
____	____	____	4. Squeeze bottle to empty contents into the rectum and colon (approximately 240 mL of solution).	
____	____	____	5. Maintain pressure on the enema container until it is withdrawn from the rectum.	
____	____	____	6. Continue same steps as with large-volume enema.	
____	____	____	7. Document procedure and observations.	

Procedure Checklists to Accompany Craven/Hirnle's Fundamentals of Nursing: Human Health and Function, third edition.

Name _____ Date _____

Unit _____ Position _____

Instructor/Evaluator _____ Position _____

Excellemt	Satisfactory	Needs Practice	*Procedure 40-3* # Inserting a Nasogastric Tube **Goal:** To decompress the stomach to relieve pressure and prevent vomiting, to deliver enteral feedings, and to provide a means to irrigate the stomach or to obtain gastric specimen.	COMMENTS
▼	▼	▼		
____	____	____	1. Identify client and explain procedure.	
____	____	____	2. Provide privacy by closing curtains or room door.	
____	____	____	3. Raise bed to high-Fowler's position, cover chest with towel, and place emesis basin nearby.	
____	____	____	4. Wash hands and put on clean gloves.	
____	____	____	5. Determine length of tubing to be inserted by measuring nasogastric tube from tip of ear lobe to tip of nose, then to tip of xiphoid process. Mark tubing with adhesive tape or note striped markings already on tube.	
____	____	____	6. Lubricate tip of tube with water-soluble lubricant.	
____	____	____	7. Gently insert tube into nostril. Advance toward posterior pharynx.	
____	____	____	8. Have client tilt head forward and encourage client to drink water slowly. Advance tube without using force as client swallows. Advance tube until desired insertion length is reached.	
____	____	____	9. Temporarily tape the tube to client's nose; then assess placement of tube:	
____	____	____	a. Aspirate gastric content with 20–50 mL syringe.	
____	____	____	b. Auscultate over epigastrium while injecting 10–20 mL air into nasogastric tube.	
____	____	____	10. If placement in stomach is not verified, untape tube, advance tube 5 cm, and repeat assessment in Step 9.	
____	____	____	11. Secure tube by taping to bridge of client's nose. Anchor tubing to client's gown.	
____	____	____	12. Clamp end of tubing or attach to suction, as ordered by health care provider.	

Excellemt ▼	Satisfactory ▼	Needs Practice ▼	*Procedure 40-3* # Inserting a Nasogastric Tube (continued)	COMMENTS
___	___	___	13. Wash hands, provide for client's comfort, and remove equipment.	
___	___	___	14. Establish and document a nursing plan for daily care of nasogastric tube:	
___	___	___	15. a. Inspect nostril for irritation.	
___	___	___	b. Cleanse nostril frequently.	
___	___	___	c. Change adhesive as required to prevent skin irritation or pressure sores on nostril from tube.	
___	___	___	d. Increase frequency of oral care because clients with nasogastric tubes often mouth breathe and may be NPO.	
___	___	___	16. Document procedure and observations.	

Procedure Checklists to Accompany Craven/Hirnle's Fundamentals of Nursing: Human Health and Function, third edition.

Name _____ Date _____

Unit _____ Position _____

Instructor/Evaluator _____ Position _____

Excellent	Satisfactory	Needs Practice	
▼	▼	▼	*Procedure 40-4* **Applying a Fecal Ostomy Pouch** **Goal:** To provide a means to contain drainage and odors from a fecal ostomy. COMMENTS
___	___	___	1. Provide privacy.
___	___	___	2. Don disposable gloves.
___	___	___	3. Gently remove old appliance. If disposable, discard. If reusable, set aside for washing.
___	___	___	4. Wash skin thoroughly around stoma with skin cleanser or soap and water.
___	___	___	5. Rinse skin thoroughly and blot dry.
___	___	___	6. Observe condition of peristomal skin, the stoma, and the sutures. Teach client to make these observations daily.
___	___	___	7. Prepare clean pouch. Measure stoma and trace circle 1/8-inch larger than stoma on adhesive paper backing. Cut stoma pattern.
___	___	___	8. Prepare skin barrier. Measure stoma and cut hole in barrier the same size as stoma. Be sure edges are rounded.
___	___	___	9. If stoma located in abdominal crease or skin is irregular, use paste barrier to fill the irregularity.
___	___	___	10. Apply protective skin barrier:
___	___	___	a. Peel paper backing off wafer and center stoma in hole.
___	___	___	b. Place on abdomen, pressing lightly over all areas of the barrier to promote adhesion with skin surfaces.
___	___	___	11. Attach drainable pouch to skin barrier. (Some equipment attaches by plastic flange that snaps in place; other models adhere through self-adherent tape that is exposed after protective paper backing is removed.) Tug gently or inspect for secure fit.
___	___	___	12. Frame every edge of the faceplate with hypoallergenic tape to provide reinforcement.

Excellent ▼	Satisfactory ▼	Needs Practice ▼	*Procedure 40-4* ## Applying a Fecal Ostomy Pouch (continued)	COMMENTS
___	___	___	13. Fold over bottom edge of pouch and clamp.	
___	___	___	14. Dispose of old appliance. Clean and store any reusable supplies.	
___	___	___	15. Wash hands.	
___	___	___	16. Document noted observations.	